HEALTH CARE IN TRANSITION

MEDICAID EXPANSION UNDER THE AFFORDABLE CARE ACT

OVERVIEW AND MISSED OPPORTUNITIES

Health Care in Transition

Additional books in this series can be found on Nova's website under the Series tab.

Additional e-books in this series can be found on Nova's website under the e-book tab.

HEALTH CARE IN TRANSITION

MEDICAID EXPANSION UNDER THE AFFORDABLE CARE ACT

OVERVIEW AND MISSED OPPORTUNITIES

GAIL NORMAN
EDITOR

nova publishers
New York

Additional color graphics may be available in the e-book version of this book.

Library of Congress Cataloging-in-Publication Data

ISBN: 978-1-63463-442-7

Published by Nova Science Publishers, Inc. † New York

CONTENTS

PREFACE

Historically, Medicaid eligibility has generally been limited to certain low-income children, pregnant women, parents of dependent children, the elderly, and individuals with disabilities; however, as of January 1, 2014, states have the option to extend Medicaid coverage to most nonelderly, low-income individuals. The Patient Protection and Affordable Care Act established 133% of the federal poverty level (FPL) as the new mandatory minimum Medicaid income eligibility level for most nonelderly individuals. This book provides an overview of the ACA Medicaid expansion, and the impact of the Supreme Court decision on the ACA Medicaid expansion. Then, the book describes who is covered under the expansion, the expansion rules, and how the expansion is financed. In addition, enrollment and expenditure estimates for the ACA Medicaid expansion are provided. The book reviews state decisions whether or not to implement the ACA Medicaid expansion, and the implications of those decisions on certain individuals, employers, and hospitals.

Chapter 1 – Federal judges and the journalists who cover them share much common ground. One clear area of mutual interest is accurate and informed coverage of federal courts. *A Journalist's Guide to the Federal Courts* is intended to assist reporters assigned to court coverage. It is the media who inform and educate the public about the courts, spark discussion and debate about their work, instill public trust and confidence in the institution and its function, and help protect judicial independence. These are worthwhile and important pursuits. There are justifiable and distinct differences between the three branches of government and the access they grant the news media. Most of the work of federal courts is performed in open court and decisions, and in most cases court filings are available on the Internet. This primer is aimed at helping reporters who cover federal appellate, district, and bankruptcy courts – the cases, the people, and the process.

Chapter 2 – This report provides an analysis of the professional qualifications and experiences of U.S. circuit court judges who are currently serving on the federal bench. Interest in the professional qualifications of those nominated to the federal judiciary has been demonstrated by Congress and others. Congressional interest in the professional experiences of those nominated by a President to the federal courts reflects, in part, the evaluative role of Congress in examining the qualifications of those who are nominated to life-tenure positions. Other organizations, such as the American Bar Association (ABA), also have an ongoing interest in the professional qualifications of those appointed to the federal judiciary. Additionally, scholars have demonstrated an interest in this topic by examining whether a relationship exists between the professional or career experiences of judges and judicial decision making.

Chapter 3 – The Affordable Care Act has expanded high-quality, affordable health insurance coverage to millions of Americans. One important way in which the Affordable Care Act is expanding coverage is by providing generous financial support to States that opt to expand Medicaid eligibility to all non-elderly individuals in families with incomes below 133 percent of the Federal Poverty Level. To date, 26 States and the District of Columbia have seized this opportunity, and since the beginning of the Affordable Care Act's first open enrollment period, 5.2 million people have gained Medicaid or Children's Health Insurance Program (CHIP) coverage in these States, a tally that will grow in the months and years ahead as Medicaid enrollment continues. In contrast, 24 States have not yet expanded Medicaid—including many of the States that would benefit most and sometimes because State legislatures have defied even their own governors—and denied health insurance coverage to millions of their citizens. Researchers at the Urban Institute estimate that, if these States do not change course, 5.7 million people will be deprived of health insurance coverage in 2016. Meanwhile, these States will forgo billions in Federal dollars that could boost their economies. This analysis uses the best evidence from the economics and health policy literatures to quantify several important consequences of States' decisions not to expand Medicaid. That evidence, which is based primarily on careful analysis of the effects of past policy decisions, is necessarily an imperfect guide to the future, and the actual effects of Medicaid expansion under the Affordable Care Act could be larger or smaller than the estimates presented below.

However, this evidence is clear that the consequences of States' decisions are far-reaching, with implications for the health and well-being of their citizens, their economies, and the economy of the Nation as a whole.

In: Medicaid Expansion …
Editor: Gail Norman
ISBN: 978-1-63463-442-7

Chapter 1

THE ACA MEDICAID EXPANSION*

Alison Mitchell

SUMMARY

Historically, Medicaid eligibility has generally been limited to certain low-income children, pregnant women, parents of dependent children, the elderly, and individuals with disabilities; however, as of January 1, 2014, states have the option to extend Medicaid coverage to most nonelderly, low-income individuals.

The Patient Protection and Affordable Care Act (ACA, P.L. 111-148 as amended) established 133% of the federal poverty level (FPL) (effectively 138% of FPL with an income disregard of 5% of FPL) as the new mandatory minimum Medicaid income eligibility level for most nonelderly individuals. On June 28, 2012, the United States Supreme Court issued its decision in *National Federation of Independent Business v. Sebelius*, finding that the enforcement mechanism for the ACA Medicaid expansion violated the Constitution, which effectively made the ACA Medicaid expansion optional for states.

If a state accepts the ACA Medicaid expansion funds, it must abide by the new expansion coverage rules. For instance, modified adjusted gross income (MAGI) counting rules are used for determining eligibility for the ACA Medicaid expansion population, and individuals covered

---

* This is an edited, reformatted and augmented version of a Congressional Research Service publication R43564, prepared for Members and Committees of Congress, dated May 23, 2014.

under the ACA Medicaid expansion are required to receive alternative benefit plan (ABP) coverage.

The ACA provides different federal Medicaid matching rates for the individuals who will gain Medicaid coverage through the ACA Medicaid expansion. The federal government's share of most Medicaid expenditures is determined according to the federal medical assistance percentage (FMAP) rate, but exceptions to the regular FMAP rate have been made for certain states, situations, populations, providers, and services. The ACA adds a few FMAP exceptions for the ACA Medicaid expansion: the "newly eligible" FMAP rate, the "expansion state" FMAP rate, and the additional FMAP increase for certain expansion states.

On January 1, 2014, when the ACA Medicaid expansion went into effect, 24 states and the District of Columbia had the ACA Medicaid expansion included as part of their Medicaid programs. Michigan implemented the expansion on April 1, 2014, and New Hampshire plans to implement the expansion on July 1, 2014. Most states implementing the ACA Medicaid expansion will do so through an expansion of their current Medicaid program. However, some states are implementing the expansion through an alternative health care delivery method, namely premium assistance.

State decisions *not* to implement the ACA Medicaid expansion could have implications for low-income individuals, large employers with low-wage workers, and hospitals. For example, most uninsured individuals with incomes under 100% of FPL will likely remain uninsured, and large employers with low-wage workers might have greater exposure to employer penalties included in the ACA. Also, Medicaid DSH allotments will be reduced by the same across the nation whether or not states implement the expansion.

INTRODUCTION

Medicaid is a means-tested entitlement program that finances the delivery of primary and acute care services, as well as long-term services and supports.[1] It is a federal-state program, and participation in Medicaid is voluntary for states, though all states and the District of Columbia choose to participate. In order to participate in Medicaid, the federal government requires states to cover certain mandatory populations and benefits, but the federal government also allows states to cover optional populations and services. Due to this flexibility, there is substantial variation among the states in terms of factors such as Medicaid eligibility, covered benefits, and provider payment rates.

Medicaid is jointly financed by the federal government and the states. States incur Medicaid costs by making payments to service providers (e.g., for doctor visits) and performing administrative activities (e.g., making eligibility determinations), and the federal government reimburses states for a share of these costs.[2] The federal government's share of a state's expenditures for most Medicaid services is called the federal medical assistance percentage (FMAP).[3] The FMAP varies by state and is inversely related to each state's per capita income. For FY2014, FMAP rates range from 50% (15 states) to 73% (Mississippi).

Historically, Medicaid eligibility has generally been limited to certain low-income children, pregnant women, parents of dependent children, the elderly, and individuals with disabilities; however, starting January 1, 2014, states have the option to extend Medicaid coverage to most nonelderly, nonpregnant adults with income up to 133% of the federal poverty (FPL). This expansion of Medicaid eligibility is one of a number of changes the Patient Protection and Affordable Care Act (ACA , P.L. 111-148 as amended) made to the Medicaid program, and it is referred to as the ACA Medicaid expansion.

This report provides an overview of the ACA Medicaid expansion, and the impact of the Supreme Court decision on the ACA Medicaid expansion. Then, the report describes who is covered under the expansion, the expansion rules, and how the expansion is financed. In addition, enrollment and expenditure estimates for the ACA Medicaid expansion are provided. Finally, the report reviews state decisions whether or not to implement the ACA Medicaid expansion, and the implications of those decisions on certain individuals, employers, and hospitals.

Medicaid Eligibility before the Expansion

A common misconception about the Medicaid program is that all low-income individuals are eligible for Medicaid. Instead, only certain low-income individuals are eligible for Medicaid coverage. To qualify, an individual must meet both categorical (i.e., must be a member of a covered group, such as children, pregnant women, parents with dependent children, the elderly, or individuals with disabilities) and financial eligibility requirements. In addition, individuals need to meet federal and state requirements regarding residency, immigration status, and documentation of U.S. citizenship.[4]

The federal Medicaid statute (Title XIX of the Social Security Act) defines a number of distinct population groups as being potentially eligible for

Medicaid coverage. Some of these populations are mandatory eligibility groups that states must cover if they choose to participate in Medicaid, while others are optional eligibility groups that states are allowed to cover if they choose to do so. In addition, states are able to provide Medicaid coverage to additional populations not listed as a mandatory or optional coverage group in statute through Section 1115 demonstration waivers.[5] Due to optional eligibility groups and the Section 1115 demonstration waivers, Medicaid eligibility varies significantly from state to state.

The bars in *Figure 1* show the federally mandated Medicaid income eligibility levels for the major population groups that were in effect prior to the implementation of the ACA Medicaid expansion. Then, the text in *Figure 1* indicates the number of states using optional eligibility groups and Section 1115 waivers to have income eligibility levels above the federally mandated level in January 2013 and the highest income eligibility level for each population.

The ACA Medicaid expansion provides states with the option to increase Medicaid eligibility to 133% of the FPL for nonelderly, nonpregnant adults. As shown in *Figure 1*, prior to the ACA, Medicaid income eligibility levels for parents with dependent children were low relative to the income eligibility levels for children and pregnant women, and adults without dependent children were not eligible for Medicaid in most states. For this reason, 70% of low-income children had Medicaid coverage, while 30% of low-income, nonelderly adults had Medicaid coverage. In addition, the uninsured rate for low-income, nonelderly adults was 42%, which was more than twice the national average of 18%.[6]

ACA Medicaid Expansion

The primary goals of ACA are to increase access to affordable health insurance for the uninsured and to make health insurance more affordable for those already covered. The ACA Medicaid expansion is one of the major insurance coverage provisions included in the law, but the ACA Medicaid expansion is just one of a few Medicaid eligibility expansions included in the ACA.[7]

The ACA Medicaid expansion (as initially enacted) established 133% of FPL as the new mandatory minimum Medicaid income eligibility level for most nonelderly, nonpregnant adults.

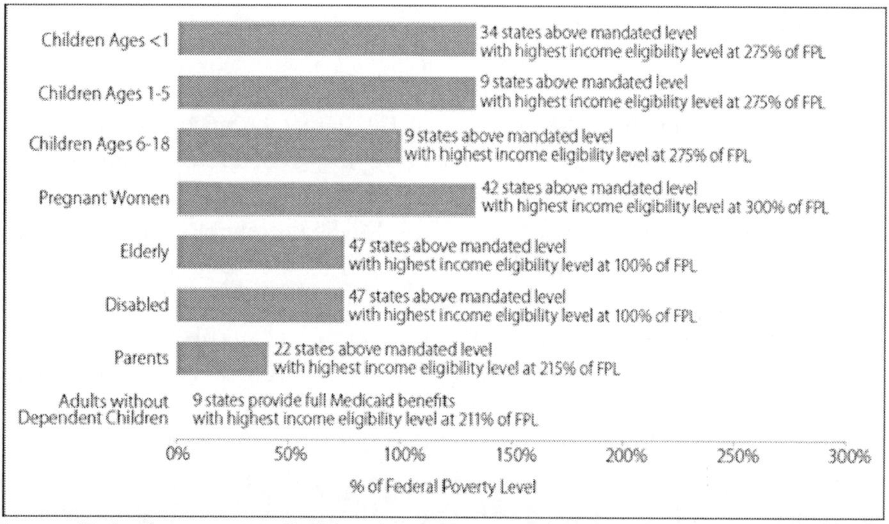

Source: Federal statute; Medicaid and CHIP Payment and Access Commission, Report to Congress on Medicaid and CHIP, March 2013, Table 110 on page 94.

Notes: As of January 1, 2014, the federally mandated Medicaid eligibility level for children ages six through 18 increased from 100% to 133% of FPL as part of the ACA but not as part of the optional ACA Medicaid expansion.

FPL: Federal poverty level.

Figure 1. Federally Mandated Medicaid Income Eligibility Criteria as a Percentage of FPL, by Major Population Category. (January 2013).

The law also specified that an income disregard in the amount of 5% of FPL be deducted from an individual's income when determining Medicaid eligibility based on the modified adjusted gross income (MAGI).[8] Thus, the upper income eligibility threshold for individuals in this new eligibility group is effectively 138% of FPL. This ACA Medicaid expansion was effective January 1, 2014 (or earlier at state option).[9]

The Supreme Court decision in *National Federation of Independent Business (NFIB) v. Sebelius* made the ACA Medicaid expansion optional rather than mandatory. In states that adopt the ACA Medicaid expansion, the three major groups of individuals gaining Medicaid coverage are adults without dependent children, parents with dependent children, and adults with disabilities. States that implement the ACA Medicaid expansion are required to follow the ACA Medicaid expansion rules. The federal government funds a vast majority of the cost for the ACA Medicaid expansion.

Supreme Court Decision

Originally, it was assumed that all states would implement the ACA Medicaid expansion in 2014 as required by statute because implementation was required in order for states to receive *any* federal Medicaid funding. However, with respect to Medicaid, the Supreme Court decision in *NFIB* addressed the issue of whether withholding Medicaid reimbursement to a state unless that state complies with the expansion of its Medicaid program exceeds Congress's enumerated powers under the Spending Clause and/or violates the Tenth Amendment. On June 28, 2012, the Supreme Court issued its decision in *NFIB*, and the Supreme Court held that the ACA Medicaid expansion violated the Constitution.[10]

The Supreme Court decision held that the federal government could not withhold payment for a state's entire Medicaid program for failure to implement the ACA Medicaid expansion. However, the federal government could withhold the funding for the ACA Medicaid expansion if a state did not implement the expansion. As a result, the Supreme Court's ruling in *NFIB* effectively made state participation in the ACA Medicaid expansion voluntary. The federal government cannot terminate federal Medicaid matching funds for a state's pre-ACA Medicaid program if a state doesn't implement the ACA Medicaid expansion.

After the Supreme Court ruling, the Centers for Medicare & Medicaid Services (CMS) issued guidance to states specifying that states have no deadline for deciding when to implement the ACA Medicaid expansion. Also, the guidance said that states that decide to implement the expansion have the ability to end the ACA Medicaid expansion at any point in time.[11]

Who Is Covered under the Expansion

The three major categories of nonelderly adults that would receive Medicaid coverage under the ACA Medicaid expansion are adults without dependent children, parents with dependent children, and adults with disabilities. Prior to the implementation of the ACA Medicaid expansion, only a few states provided Medicaid coverage to adults without dependent children, and in general, the Medicaid income eligibility level for parents and adults with disabilities was significantly lower than 133% of FPL (i.e., the ACA Medicaid expansion eligibility level).

Adults without Dependent Children

Prior to the ACA, adults without dependent children were not included in the federal statute as either a mandatory or an optional Medicaid coverage group. However, states were able to provide Medicaid coverage to these adults through Section 1115 demonstration waivers or state-funded programs.

As of January 2013, eight states (Arizona, Colorado, Connecticut, Delaware, Hawaii, Minnesota, New York, and Vermont)[12] and the District of Columbia provided full Medicaid coverage to adults without dependent children, and only two of these states and the District of Columbia covered adults without dependent children up to at least 133% of FPL. In addition, 18 states[13] provided Medicaid coverage with limited benefits to adults without dependent children.[14]

For most states, a significant portion of the population that would gain Medicaid coverage through the implementation of the ACA Medicaid expansion would be adults without dependent children. See *Figure A-1* for state-by-state Medicaid income eligibility levels for nonelderly adults without dependent children as of January 1, 2014.

Parents

Under Section 1931 of the Social Security Act, states are required to provide Medicaid coverage for parents (and their dependent children), at a minimum, at the Aid to Families with Dependent Children (AFDC) eligibility levels in place on July 16, 1996.[15] This federally mandated eligibility threshold varies by state but averages 41% of FPL.[16]

Section 1931 of the Social Security Act also gives states the option to cover parents with incomes above the 1996 minimum levels and most states do. As of January 2013, 12 states[17] provided full Medicaid coverage for parents of dependent children with incomes at or above 133% of FPL, and 13 states[18] provided Medicaid coverage with limited benefits to parents of dependent children with incomes of 133% of FPL or higher.[19]

In most states, the ACA Medicaid expansion would provide Medicaid coverage to a significant number of parents with dependent children. See *Figure A-2* for state-by-state Medicaid income eligibility levels for parents with dependent children as of January 1, 2014.

Adults with Disabilities

The major Medicaid eligibility pathway for nonelderly, disabled individuals is based on the program rules for the Supplemental Security Income (SSI) program. Federal law requires states to provide Medicaid coverage to recipients of SSI. The income eligibility threshold for SSI translates to 74% of the FPL in 2014.[20] However, Section 209(b) of the Social Security Amendments of 1972 (P.L. 92-603) gave states the option to use Medicaid eligibility criteria for adults with disabilities with income and resources thresholds that are more restrictive than SSI but no more restrictive than those in effect on January 1, 1972.[21] Therefore, in 209(b) states, receipt of SSI does not guarantee eligibility for Medicaid.

States also have the option to provide Medicaid coverage to nonelderly adults with disabilities through other optional eligibility pathways, such as the poverty level, medically needy, and special income level.[22]

Prior to the ACA Medicaid expansion, all states had Medicaid income eligibility thresholds for nonelderly adults with disabilities below 133% of FPL. As a result, the implementation of the ACA Medicaid expansion would provide a significant increase in the Medicaid income eligibility level for nonelderly adults with disabilities. See *Figure A-3* for state-by-state Medicaid income eligibility levels for nonelderly adults with disabilities as of January 1, 2014.

ACA Medicaid Expansion Rules

While the ACA Medicaid expansion makes additional nonelderly adults eligible for Medicaid, the requirements for the ACA Medicaid expansion vary from other aspects of the program. If a state accepts the ACA Medicaid expansion funds, it must abide by the new expansion coverage rules. For instance, MAGI counting rules are used for determining eligibility for the ACA Medicaid expansion population,[23] and individuals covered under the ACA Medicaid expansion are required to receive alternative benefit plan (ABP) coverage.

MAGI Income Counting Rules

As of January 1, 2014, the MAGI counting rules are used in determining eligibility for most of Medicaid's nonelderly populations, including the ACA Medicaid expansion. MAGI is defined as the Internal Revenue Code's adjusted gross income (AGI, which reflects a number of deductions, including trade and business deductions, losses from sale of property, and alimony payments) increased (if applicable) by tax-exempt interest and income earned by U.S. citizens or residents living abroad.[24]

Under the MAGI counting rules, the state looks at the individual's MAGI, deduct 5%, which the law provides as a standard disregard, and compare that income to the MAGI income standards set by each state in coordination with CMS.[25]

ABP Coverage

The ACA mandates the individuals gaining Medicaid coverage through the ACA Medicaid expansion receive Medicaid benefits through ABPs, which are a Medicaid benefit structure that has different requirements than the traditional Medicaid benefits.[26] In general, ABP coverage may be less generous than traditional Medicaid coverage but more generous than most private health insurance coverage. ABPs may cover fewer benefits than traditional Medicaid, but there are some requirements, such as coverage of family planning and transportation services that private insurance generally does not cover.[27] As a result, an adult with disabilities may have access to different coverage through the ACA Medicaid expansion eligibility pathway (i.e., eligible for Medicaid based solely on their low-income status) than the adults with disabilities that have Medicaid coverage through the SSI eligibility pathway (i.e., eligible for Medicaid based on being low-income and disabled).[28] However, during the application process, states must identify those who are medically frail and offer them a choice of ABP or traditional Medicaid benefits as their ABP coverage.[29]

Financing

The ACA provides different federal Medicaid matching rates for the individuals that will gain Medicaid coverage through the ACA Medicaid expansion. The federal government's share of most Medicaid expenditures is determined according to the FMAP rate,[30] but exceptions to the regular FMAP rate have been made for certain states, situations, populations, providers, and services. The ACA adds a few FMAP exceptions for the ACA Medicaid expansion: the "newly eligible" FMAP rate, the "expansion state" FMAP rate, and the additional FMAP increase for certain expansion states.

"Newly Eligible" FMAP Rates

The "newly eligible" FMAP rate is used to reimburse states for the Medicaid expenditures for "newly eligible" individuals who gained Medicaid eligibility due to the ACA Medicaid expansion. The "newly eligible" individuals are defined as nonelderly, nonpregnant adults with family income below 133% FPL who would not have been eligible for Medicaid in the state as of December 1, 2009 (or were eligible under a waiver but not enrolled because of limits or caps on waiver enrollment). States will receive 100% FMAP rate (i.e., full federal financing) for the cost of providing Medicaid coverage to "newly eligible" individuals, from 2014 through 2016. For "newly eligible" individuals, the FMAP rate will phase down to 95% in 2017, 94% in 2018, 93% in 2019, and 90% afterward (*Table 1*).

Federal statute specifies the "newly eligible" FMAP rate for each year, which means the "newly eligible" FMAP rates are available for these specific years regardless of when a state implements the ACA Medicaid expansion. For instance, if a state implements the ACA Medicaid expansion in 2018, then that state will receive a "newly eligible" FMAP rate of 94% in 2018, 93% in 2019, and 90% afterward.

Table 1. FMAP Rates for ACA Medicaid Expansion

	2014	2015	2016	2017	2018	2019	2020+
"Newly eligible"	100%	100%	100%	95%	94%	93%	90%
Adults in all States							
Certain Individuals	75%-	80%-	85%-	86%-	90%-	93%	90%
in "Expansion states"	92%	93%	95%	93%	93%		

Source: Prepared by CRS.

Notes: For the calculation of the "expansion state" FMAP rates, the lower bound is for a state with a regular FMAP rate of 50% (which is the statutory minimum), and the upper bound is for a state with a regular FMAP rate of 83% (which is the statutory maximum).

"Expansion State" FMAP Rates

As mentioned earlier, prior to the ACA some states provided Medicaid coverage to adults without dependent children and to parents with incomes above the threshold for the Section 1931 pathway using Section 1115 waivers. As a result, these states have few or no individuals who will qualify for the "newly eligible" FMAP rate. As of 2014, these states receive an increased FMAP rate, which is referred to as the "expansion state" FMAP rate.

This definition of expansion state was established prior to the Supreme Court decision making ACA Medicaid expansion optional for states. In this context, expansion state refers to states that had already implemented (or partially implemented) the ACA Medicaid expansion at the time the ACA was enacted. Specifically, "expansion states" are defined as those that, as of March

23, 2010 (ACA's enactment date), provided health benefits coverage meeting certain criteria[31] statewide to parents with dependent children and adults without dependent children at least through 100% of FPL.[32] As of early December 2013, the Centers for Medicare & Medicaid Services (CMS) determined the following states met the definition of "expansion state" and would be eligible for the "expansion state" FMAP rate if the state implements the ACA Medicaid expansion: Arizona, Delaware, District of Columbia, Hawaii, Maine, Massachusetts, Minnesota, New York, Pennsylvania, Vermont, and Washington.[33]

The "expansion state" FMAP rate is available for individuals in "expansion states" that have implemented the ACA Medicaid expansion[34] who were eligible for Medicaid on March 23, 2010 and are in the new eligibility group for nonelderly, nonpregnant adults at or below 133% FPL. The formula[35] used to calculate the "expansion state" FMAP rates is based on a state's regular FMAP rate, so the "expansion state" FMAP rates will vary from state to state until CY2019, at which point the "newly eligible" FMAP rates and the "expansion state" FMAP rates will both be equal (see *Table 1)*.

"Expansion states" are not excluded from receiving the "newly eligible" FMAP rates. Populations in an "expansion state" that meet the definition for the "newly eligible" FMAP rate will receive the "newly eligible" FMAP rate. For example, an "expansion state" that prior to the ACA provided Medicaid coverage to nonelderly adults without dependent children and parents with dependent children up to 100% FPL, will receive the higher "newly eligible" FMAP rate for individuals between 100% and 133% FPL if it implements the ACA Medicaid expansion. Also, "expansion states" will receive the "newly eligible" FMAP rate for individuals who received limited Medicaid benefits prior to the expansion. In addition, "expansion states" that provided state-funded health benefits coverage will receive the "newly eligible" FMAP rate for individuals previously covered by the state-only program.[36]

Additional FMAP Increase for Certain "Expansion States"

During 2014 and 2015, an FMAP rate increase of 2.2 percentage points is available for "expansion states" that (1) the Secretary of the Department of Health & Human Services (HHS) determines will not receive any FMAP rate increase for "newly eligible" individuals and (2) have not been approved to use Medicaid disproportionate share hospital (DSH) funds to pay for the cost of health coverage under a waiver in effect as of July 2009.[37] The FMAP rate increase applies to those individuals who are not "newly eligible" individuals, such as nonelderly adults without dependent children and parents with dependent children up to 100% FPL because they would have been eligible for Medicaid prior to the implementation of the ACA Medicaid expansion in an "expansion state." Vermont is the only state that has been confirmed as meeting the criteria for the additional FMAP increase for certain "expansion states."

Enrollment and Expenditure Estimates

The ACA Medicaid expansion is expected to significantly increase Medicaid enrollment and federal Medicaid expenditures.

In terms of enrollment, the Congressional Budget Office (CBO) estimates the insurance coverage provisions from the ACA will increase Medicaid and the State Children's Health Insurance Program (CHIP) enrollment of nonelderly individuals by 13 million in FY2024.[38] A vast majority of the increase in enrollment for Medicaid and CHIP is due to the ACA Medicaid expansion, but enrollment is also impacted by other provisions, such as the expansion of Medicaid eligibility for foster care children and children ages six to 18.

Figure 2 shows the year-by-year estimates of the effects of the ACA insurance coverage provisions on Medicaid and CHIP enrollment. Even without all states participating in the ACA Medicaid expansion, the ACA insurance coverage provisions are expected to increase Medicaid and CHIP enrollment for nonelderly individuals by more than 25% in each year after FY2015.[39]

Regardless of whether a state decides to implement the ACA Medicaid expansion or not, all states are expected to experience an increase in Medicaid enrollment, due to the "woodwork" effect. This is the term for uninsured individuals who, without the expansion are eligible for Medicaid, but decide to enroll in Medicaid due to increased media attention and outreach efforts associated with the ACA. The impact of the woodwork effect depends on the percentage of a state's population that is eligible but not enrolled in Medicaid. Nationally, an estimated 7.3 million to 9.0 million uninsured children and adults were eligible but not enrolled in Medicaid prior to the implementation of the expansion.[40]

Figure 3 shows the annual estimated federal budgetary effect of the ACA insurance coverage provisions on Medicaid and CHIP outlays compared to estimated Medicaid and CHIP outlays without the ACA insurance coverage provisions.

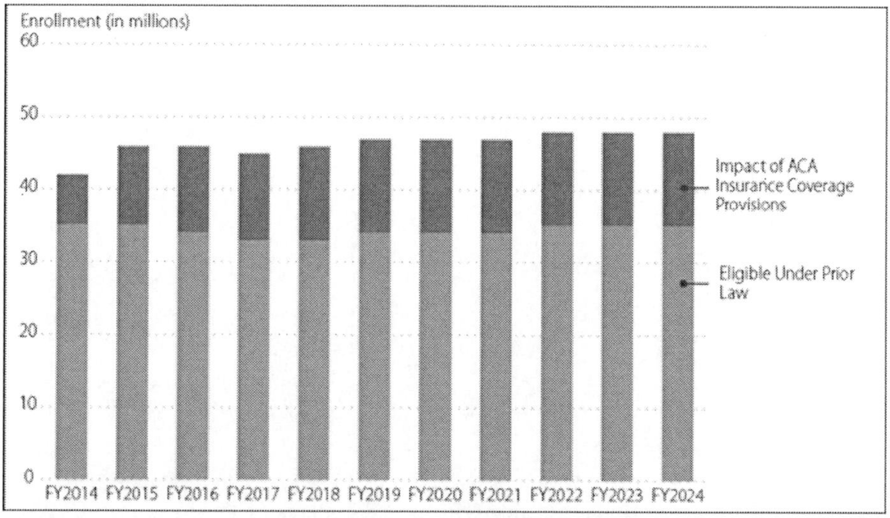

Source: Congressional Budget Office, Updated Estimates of the Insurance Coverage Provisions of the Affordable Care Act, April 2014.

Notes: Figure reflects average enrollment over the course of a year.

Figure 2. Estimated Effects of ACA Insurance Coverage Provisions on Medicaid and CHIP Enrollment for Nonelderly Individuals. (FY2014 to FY2024).

A vast majority of the federal expenditures for the Medicaid and CHIP insurance coverage provisions are due to the ACA Medicaid expansion, but these expenditures also include other provisions, such as the expansion of Medicaid eligibility for foster care children and children ages six to 18. From FY2015 through FY2024, CBO estimates the ACA Medicaid and CHIP insurance coverage provisions will increase Medicaid and CHIP outlays by almost 23%.[41]

The federal government will be covering a vast majority (94%) of the cost of the ACA Medicaid and CHIP insurance coverage provisions. CBO estimates these provisions will increase federal Medicaid and CHIP outlays by a total of $792 billion from FY2015 through FY2024, while the state cost of these provisions is estimated to be $46 billion over the same period of time.[42]

The potential impact of the ACA Medicaid expansion varies significantly from state to state. Medicaid enrollment and expenditures are estimated to increase at varying rates from state to state due to the current variation in states' Medicaid income eligibility levels for nonelderly adults and state demographics.

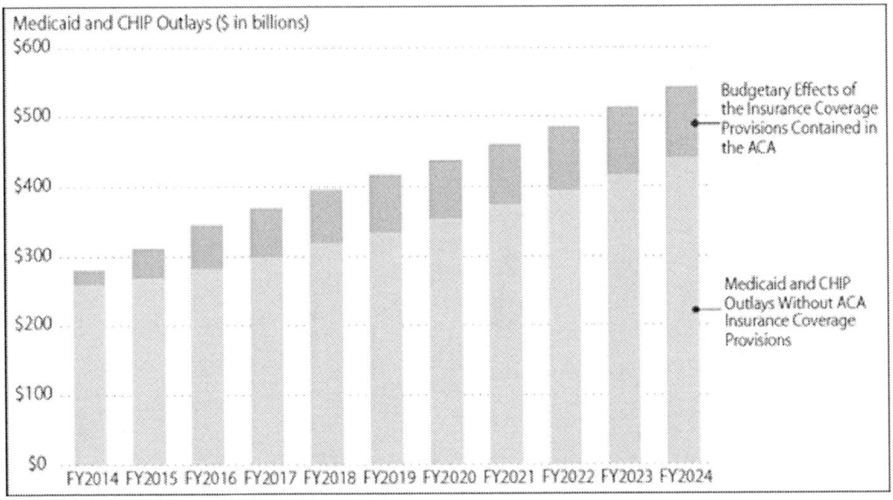

Source: Congressional Budget Office, Updated Estimates of the Insurance Coverage Provisions of the Affordable Care Act, April 2014; Congressional Budget Office, Detail of Spending and Enrollment for Medicaid for CBO's April 2014 Baseline, April 2014; Congressional Budget Office, Detail of Spending and Enrollment for Children's Health Insurance Program for CBO's April 2014 Baseline, April 2014.

Notes: Federal Medicaid expenditures excludes expenditures for disproportionate share hospital payments, Vaccines for Children, and administration.

Figure 3. Estimated Federal Medicaid and CHIP Outlays for the ACA Insurance Coverage Provisions Compared to Outlays Without the ACA Insurance Coverage Provisions. (FY2014 to FY2024).

See *Table B-1* for state-by-state estimates of the potential impact of the ACA Medicaid expansion on Medicaid expenditures and enrollment.[43]

State Decisions

On January 1, 2014, when the ACA Medicaid expansion went into effect, 24 states and the District of Columbia included the expansion as part of their Medicaid programs. Michigan implemented the expansion on April 1, 2014, and New Hampshire plans to implement the expansion on July 1, 2014.[44] See *Figure 4* for a map of the states that have and have not decided to implement the ACA Medicaid expansion as of May 21, 2014. In five of the states that have *not* expanded (Indiana, Missouri, Pennsylvania, Utah, and Virginia), the ACA Medicaid expansion is currently being debated.[45]

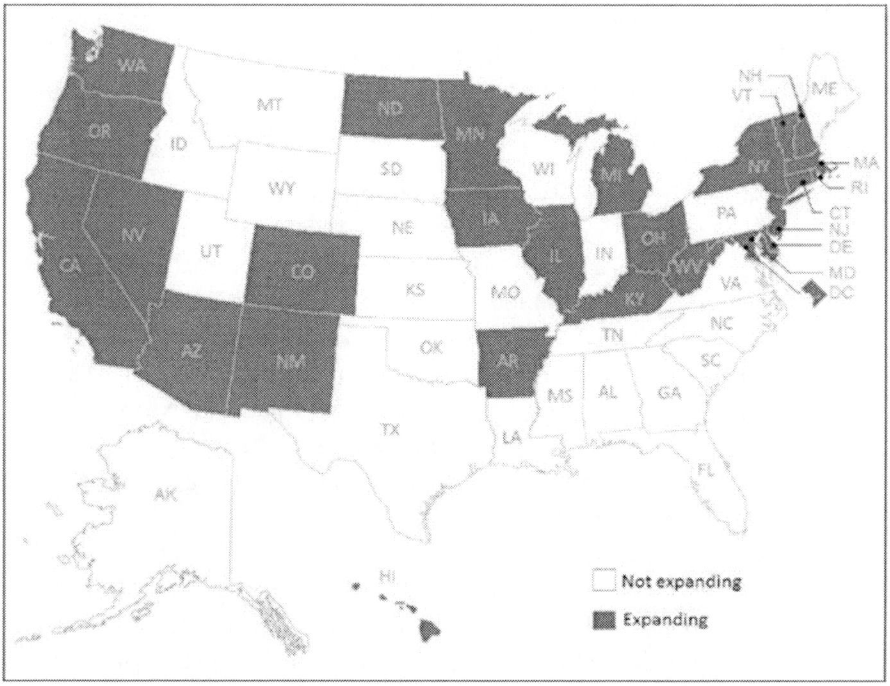

Source: States' decisions are based on CRS's monitoring of state activity through media outlets and state tracking of decisions done by CMS, State Refor(u)m, the Kaiser Family Foundation, the Advisory Board Company, and Avalere.

Note: Most states implemented the expansion on January 1, 2014, but Michigan implemented the expansion on April 1, 2014 and New Hampshire plans to implement the ACA Medicaid expansion on July 1, 2014.

Figure 4. State Decisions Whether to Implement the ACA Medicaid Expansion. (As of May 21, 2014).

While there are some exceptions, most of the states that have implemented the ACA Medicaid expansion tend to have low rates of uninsured individuals (relative to the national average) and traditionally have provided Medicaid coverage to more nonelderly adults through relatively higher Medicaid income eligibility levels. Also, in general, the states that have *not* implemented the ACA Medicaid expansion have relatively higher rates of uninsured and traditionally have covered fewer nonelderly adults under Medicaid.[46]

Since states are able to implement or discontinue the expansion at any time, the status of the ACA Medicaid expansion in states remains uncertain. State laws must be enacted and funds appropriated in order to implement or discontinue a Medicaid expansion decision.[47] As a result, states' decisions regarding the expansion generally occur during the legislative sessions, which generally occur during the first half of the calendar year.

The following are some examples of the ACA Medicaid expansion debates in state legislatures so far this year:

- *Arkansas* (expanded)—Some state lawmakers withdrew support for the expansion which could have led to a discontinuation of the expansion in Arkansas. However, funding for the expansion was eventually provided in the state's budget for state FY2015.[48]
- *New Hampshire* (expanded)—A bipartisan group of state Senators came to an agreement about implementing the expansion. The New Hampshire legislature approved the ACA Medicaid expansion March 25, 2014, and the Governor signed the bill on March 27, 2014.[49]
- *Utah* (expansion under debate)—The Republican governor has decided to support the expansion.[50]
- *Virginia* (expansion under debate)—The debate about the expansion has been renewed with the new Democratic governor pushing for the expansion. A special legislative session began on March 24, 2014 in order to pass the budget with one of the major sticking points being whether or not to implement the ACA Medicaid expansion.[51]

States have chosen *not* to implement the ACA Medicaid expansion for various reasons, including because they view the expansion as unaffordable to the state and the Medicaid program as "broken."[52] However, the ACA Medicaid expansion has become more palatable for some states with CMS' approval of Arkansas' proposal to implement the ACA Medicaid expansion using the "private option," which provides premium assistance for Medicaid enrollees to purchase health insurance through the health insurance exchange.

Alternative Delivery Models

Most states implementing the ACA Medicaid expansion will do so through an expansion of their current Medicaid program. However, some states are implementing the expansion through alternative health care delivery models, such as premium assistance[53] and health savings accounts.[54]

Premium Assistance

The concept of the premium assistance option for the ACA Medicaid expansion was initiated by Arkansas in February 2013. The premium assistance option was Democratic Governor Beebe's compromise approach to garner support for the Medicaid expansion among the Republican-led legislature.[55] Under the Arkansas proposal, the state would use premium assistance to purchase health insurance coverage under the qualified health plans offered through the health insurance exchanges.[56] HHS approved Arkansas' Section 1115 demonstration waiver for the premium assistance option on September 27, 2013.[57]

Iowa is also using the premium assistance model for its ACA Medicaid expansion, and Iowa's Section 1115 demonstration waiver was approved on December 10, 2013.[58] New Hampshire adopted a version of the ACA Medicaid expansion that utilizes premium assistance,[59] and CMS is currently considering a waiver proposal from Pennsylvania that would use premium assistance.[60] Lawmakers in other states, such as Florida and Utah, have expressed interest in the premium assistance option.[61]

Premium assistance is not a new concept for Medicaid coverage. States have several options to pay premiums for adults and children to purchase coverage through private group health plans, and in some cases individual plans. States may pursue premium assistance as a state plan option without a waiver. However, most states are seeking waivers to use premium assistance for their ACA Medicaid expansion because states want to implement the premium assistance in a way not permitted through a state plan amendment.[62] For instance, Arkansas and Iowa wanted to mandate enrollment in their premium assistance programs, and Pennsylvania and Utah are pursuing the inclusion of work requirements in their Section 1115 waivers for the ACA Medicaid expansion.

HHS has stated that it will consider approving a limited number of Section 1115 demonstrations to provide premium assistance to implement the ACA Medicaid expansion through the purchase of health insurance through the health insurance exchanges.[63] CMS intends to use the results of those waivers to inform design of the state innovation waivers[64] that start in 2017.[65]

Health Savings Accounts

Michigan received CMS approval for a Section 1115 waiver to implement the ACA Medicaid expansion on December 30, 2013, and the waiver includes a provision using health savings accounts. Specifically, in Michigan, Medicaid enrollees gaining Medicaid coverage through the ACA Medicaid expansion with incomes between 100% and 138% of FPL are required to make income-based contributions to health savings accounts, which are called MI Health Accounts.[66] The details of the MI Health Accounts are still being worked out, but in general, the funding in the account will be used as the first source of payment for Medicaid costs. When the funding in the account is exhausted, the Medicaid program pays for covered services in the same manner as traditional Medicaid.[67]

In addition, the governor of Indiana is pursuing a Section 1115 demonstration waiver to implement the ACA Medicaid expansion under the Health Indiana Plan, which is a delivery model that Indiana currently uses for part of its Medicaid program.[68] Since 2008, Indiana has had a Section 1115 demonstration waiver to use Medicaid funds to provide Medicaid coverage to previously uninsured low-income adults under the Health Indiana Plan, which is a benefit package modeled after a high-deductible health plan and health savings account.[69]

States *Not* Implementing the Expansion

State decisions *not* to implement the ACA Medicaid expansion could have implications for low-income individuals, large employers with low wage workers, and hospitals. The decision for a state to opt out of the ACA Medicaid expansion is expected to increase the number of individuals in that state receiving premium tax credits and cost-sharing subsidies and create a coverage gap for individuals not eligible for those credits and subsidies. In addition, states' decisions *not* to implement the expansion may increase the number of ACA employer penalties in that state, and reduce the Medicaid DSH reduction for that state.

Low-Income Individuals

Even if a state does *not* implement the ACA Medicaid expansion, some of the individuals that would have been covered by the Medicaid expansion may still gain health insurance coverage under the ACA health insurance coverage provisions. The ACA provides premium tax credits to individuals with household income between 100% and 400% of FPL who do not have access to minimum essential coverage, and these individuals with income between 100% and 250% FPL could be eligible for cost-sharing subsidies.[70] As a result, most uninsured individuals with incomes between 100% and 133% of FPL living in states that decide *not* to implement the ACA Medicaid expansion may become eligible for premium tax credits and cost-sharing subsidies to purchase insurance through the health insurance exchanges. However, most uninsured individuals with incomes under 100% of FPL living in states that decide *not* to implement the ACA Medicaid expansion will likely remain uninsured, because these individuals are not eligible for premium tax credits or the cost-sharing subsidies to purchase health insurance through the exchanges. However, legal permanent residents within their first five years in the country are eligible for premium tax credits with incomes ranging from zero up to 400% of FPL.[71]

For this reason, after the Supreme Court decision, some states were initially interested in implementing a partial ACA Medicaid expansion rather than the full Medicaid expansion. Under the partial Medicaid expansion, Medicaid eligibility would be increased to all nonelderly individuals up to 100% of FPL rather than to 133% of FPL, because premium tax credits and cost-sharing subsidies would be available to individuals above 100% of FPL. However, CMS informed states that the 100% federal funding for 2014 through 2016 would not be available to states that implement a partial expansion. CMS said if states wish to implement the partial expansion, they could do so and receive their regular federal Medicaid matching rate through 2016, and at that point, CMS will consider Section 1115 Medicaid demonstrations with the enhanced federal matching rates.[72]

The ACA was supposed to provide health coverage for all low income individuals by providing Medicaid coverage to the individuals with the lowest incomes and providing premium tax credits and cost-sharing subsidies for coverage through the exchanges to low-income individuals with incomes above Medicaid eligibility levels. However, the Supreme Court's decision making the Medicaid expansion optional for states has created a coverage gap in states that have *not* implemented the Medicaid expansion. Nearly five million uninsured adults are estimated to be in the coverage gap resulting from states' decisions *not* to implement the ACA Medicaid expansion, which means these five million individuals have incomes above their states' Medicaid eligibility levels and below the lower income limit for premium tax credits and cost-sharing subsidies for exchange coverage.[73] *Figure A-1*, *Figure A-2*, and *Figure A-3* show the coverage gaps in states for adults without dependent children, parents, and adults with disabilities (respectively).

Large Employers with Low-Wage Workers

Large employers with low-wage workers in states that do *not* implement the ACA Medicaid expansion might have greater exposure to employer penalties included in the ACA when the penalty goes into effect in 2015.[74] The

ACA imposes penalties on "large" employers[75] if at least one of their full-time employees obtains a premium credit through the exchange. Individuals who are not offered employer-sponsored coverage and who are not eligible for Medicaid or other programs may be eligible for premium tax credits for coverage through an exchange. As mentioned above, to receive premium tax credits, individuals must have income of at least 100% and up to 400% of FPL.

In states that do *not* implement the ACA Medicaid expansion, large employers with low income workers could be at greater risk of paying the ACA employer penalty. That is because more low-income workers could qualify for premium tax credits.[76]

Hospitals

The Medicaid statute requires states to make DSH payments to hospitals treating large numbers of low-income patients. This is intended to recognize the disadvantaged financial situation of those hospitals because low-income patients are more likely to be uninsured or Medicaid enrollees. Hospitals often do not receive payment for services rendered to uninsured patients, and Medicaid provider payment rates are generally lower than the rates paid by Medicare and private insurance.[77]

The federal government provides each state an annual DSH allotment, which is the maximum amount of federal matching funds that each state can claim for Medicaid DSH payments. The ACA included a provision directing the Secretary of HHS to make aggregate reductions because the ACA health insurance coverage provisions would reduce the need for Medicaid DSH payments. The ACA Medicaid DSH reductions have been amended a few times since the ACA, but under current law, the Medicaid DSH allotments will be reduced for the years FY2017 through FY2024.

Hospitals in states that are *not* expanding Medicaid are concerned because Medicaid DSH allotments will be reduced without regard to whether or not states implement the expansion. If a state implements the expansion, uncompensated care for hospitals should decline along with the DSH allotments (though not proportionally). However, if a state chooses *not* to implement the expansion, the demand for uncompensated hospital care is expected to persist but the amount of Medicaid DSH payments hospitals receive to subsidize such care may be reduced.[78] As a result, hospitals have been encouraging states to implement the ACA Medicaid expansion in order to reduce uncompensated care for hospitals. Even though Medicaid provider rates are generally lower than the rates paid by private insurance or Medicare, hospitals are likely better off with payment for a Medicaid patient than no payment for an uninsured patient.

APPENDIX A. STATES' CURRENT MEDICAID INCOME ELIGIBILITY LEVELS

The three major categories of nonelderly adults that would receive Medicaid coverage under the ACA Medicaid expansion are adults without dependent children, parents with dependent children, and adults with disabilities. Prior to the implementation of the ACA Medicaid expansion, only a few states provided Medicaid coverage to adults without dependent children, and in general, the Medicaid income eligibility level for parents and disabled adults was significantly lower than 133% of FPL (i.e., the ACA Medicaid expansion eligibility level).

State-by-state Medicaid income eligibility levels and private health insurance exchange eligibility for subsidized coverage for nonelderly adults without dependent children, parents with dependent children, and nonelderly adults with disabilities as of January 1, 2014 are provided in *Figure A-1*, *Figure A-2*, and *Figure A-3* (respectively).

These figures show the coverage gaps in states, which means individuals with incomes that fall in the coverage gap do not have access to full Medicaid coverage or exchange subsidized coverage. States that have implemented the ACA Medicaid expansion do not have coverage gaps, while most states that have *not* implemented the expansion have coverage gaps for all three populations.

Figure A-1 shows the coverage for adults without dependent children. Most states that have implemented the ACA Medicaid expansion provide Medicaid eligibility up to 133% FPL (effectively 138% FPL with the 5% income disregard). Of the states that have implemented the expansion, only the District of Columbia and Minnesota have higher income eligibility levels at 210% FPL (effectively 215% FPL) and 200% FPL (effectively 205% FPL), respectively. Except for Wisconsin, the states that have *not* implemented the expansion do not have Medicaid coverage for adults without dependent children. Wisconsin provides Medicaid coverage to adults without dependent children up to 95% FPL (effectively 100% FPL).

Figure A-2 shows the coverage for parents with dependent children. All states provide Medicaid coverage to this population through the mandatory

Medicaid eligibility pathway of Section 1931 coverage, which requires states to provide Medicaid coverage for parents (and their dependent children), at a minimum, at the Aid to Families with Dependent Children (AFDC) eligibility levels in place on July 16, 1996. Section 1931 of the Social Security Act also gives states the option to cover parents with incomes above the 1996 minimum levels and most states do. Under Section 1931 coverage, parents receive traditional Medicaid coverage. The income eligibility level for Section 1931 coverage is less than 133% FPL for most states.

For states that have implemented the ACA Medicaid expansion and did not have Medicaid coverage for parents up to 133% FPL (effectively 138% FPL), parents with incomes above the pre-expansion level up to 133% FPL (effectively 138% FPL) receive coverage under the expansion rules (e.g., alternative benefit plan coverage).

Except for Maine and Wisconsin, the states that have *not* implemented the expansion have coverage gaps for parents with dependent children between the upper bound of their Section 1931 coverage and 100% FPL when most of these parents are eligible for subsidized coverage through the exchange. Maine and Wisconsin provide Medicaid coverage to parents with dependent children up to 100% FPL (effectively 105% FPL) and 95% FPL (effectively 100% FPL), respectively.

Figure A-3 shows coverage for adults with disabilities. All states provide Medicaid coverage to adults with disabilities through mandatory Medicaid coverage for recipients of SSI or through optional eligibility pathways, such as Section 209(b), poverty level, medically needy, and special income level. Under these eligibility pathways, adults with disabilities receive traditional Medicaid benefits.[79] In all states, the Medicaid income eligibility levels for adults with disabilities under these eligibility pathways are significantly less than 100% FPL.

For states that have implemented the ACA Medicaid expansion, adults with disabilities with incomes above the pre-expansion level up to 133% FPL (effectively 138% FPL) receive coverage under the expansion rules (e.g., alternative benefit plan coverage).

The states that have *not* implemented the expansion have coverage gaps for adults with disabilities between the upper bound of their Medicaid coverage for adults with disabilities and 100% FPL when most of these adults are eligible for subsidized coverage through the exchange.

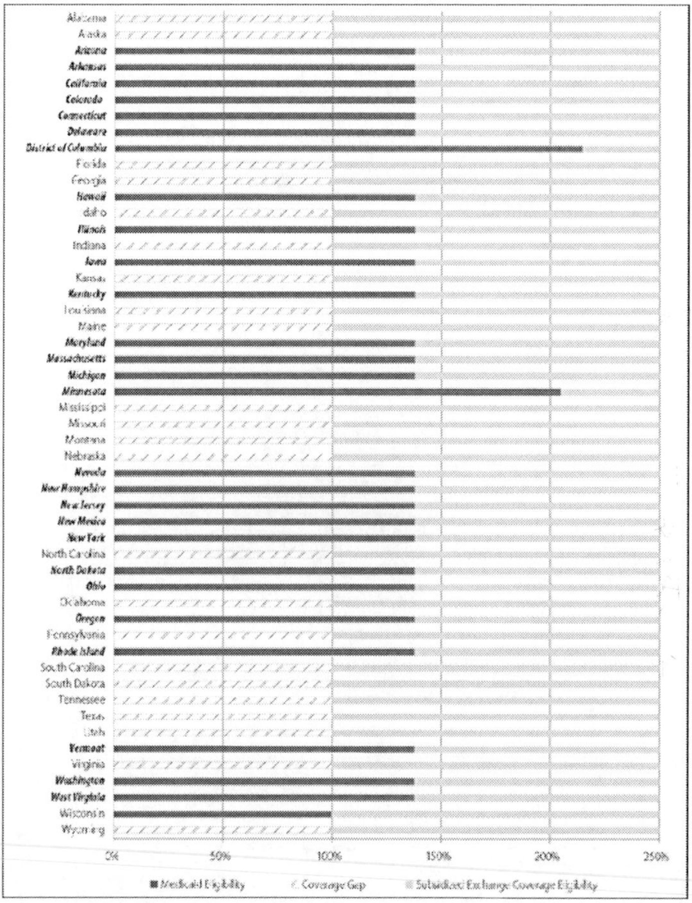

Source: Centers for Medicare & Medicaid Services, "State Medicaid and CHIP Income Eligibility Standards Effective January 1, 2014," October 24, 2013; Medicaid and CHIP Payment and Access Commission, Report to Congress on Medicaid and CHIP, March 2013, Table 110 on page 94.

Note: States in bold are states that have decided to implement the ACA Medicaid expansion. Most states implemented the expansion on January 1, 2014, but Michigan implemented the expansion on April 1, 2014 and New Hampshire plans to implement the ACA Medicaid expansion on July 1, 2014.

The "Medicaid Eligibility" category could either be the ACA Medicaid expansion implemented through state plan rules or coverage provided through a Section 1115 waiver.

Individuals with incomes that fall in the "Coverage Gap" category do not have access to full Medicaid coverage or exchange subsidized coverage.

"Subsidized Exchange Coverage Eligibility" is available to individuals with household incomes from 100% FPL through 400% FPL. The ACA provides premium tax credits to individuals with household income between 100% and 400% of FPL who do not have access to minimum essential coverage, and these individuals with income between 100% and 250% FPL could be eligible for cost-sharing subsidies.

FPL: Federal poverty level. In 2014, the federal poverty level (100% of FPL) is $11,670 for an individual and $4,060 for each additional family member in the lower 48 states and the District of Columbia.

Figure A-1. State-by-State Medicaid and Exchange Subsidized Coverage Income Eligibility Levels for Adults without Dependent Children up to 250% of FPL.(As of January 1, 2014).

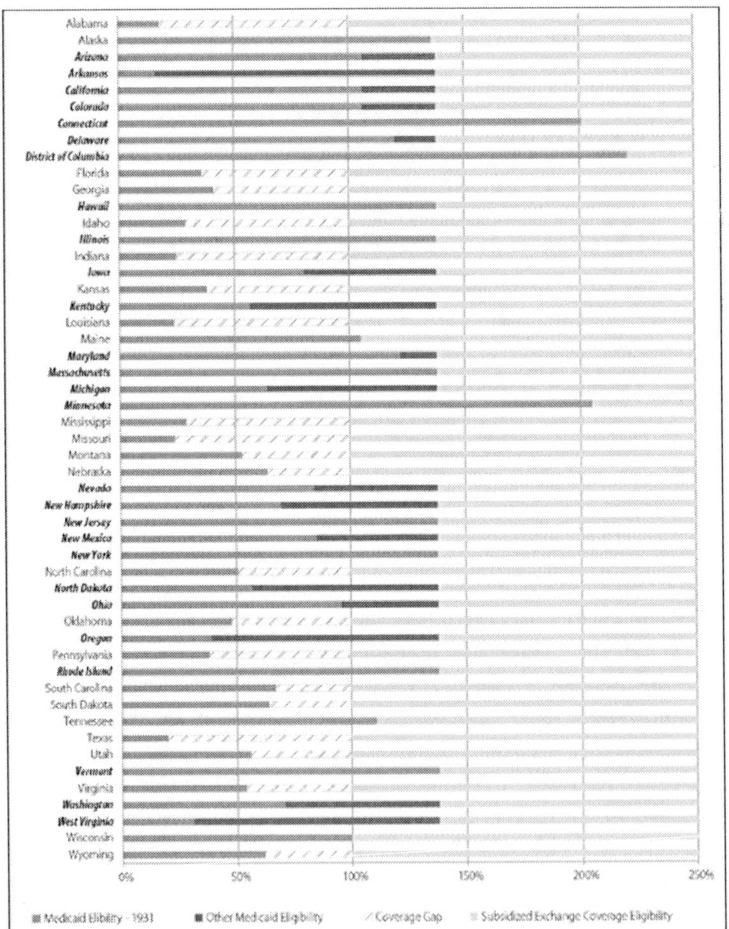

Source: Centers for Medicare & Medicaid Services, "State Medicaid and CHIP Income Eligibility Standards Effective January 1, 2014," October 24, 2013; Medicaid and

CHIP Payment and Access Commission, Report to Congress on Medicaid and CHIP, March 2013, Table 110 on page 94.

Note: States in bold are states that have decided to implement the ACA Medicaid expansion. Most states implemented the expansion on January 1, 2014, but Michigan implemented the expansion on April 1, 2014 and New Hampshire plans to implement the ACA Medicaid expansion on July 1, 2014.

Under Section 1931 of the Social Security Act, states are required to provide Medicaid coverage for parents (and their dependent children), at a minimum, at the Aid to Families with Dependent Children (AFDC) eligibility levels in place on July 16, 1996. Section 1931 of the Social Security Act also gives states the option to cover parents with incomes above the 1996 minimum levels and most states do. The "Medicaid Eligibility - 1931" category is the Medicaid income eligibility level for parents as of January 2014 for states that haven't implemented the ACA Medicaid expansion and the Medicaid income eligibility level as of January 2013 for states that have implemented the ACA Medicaid expansion. Most of the parents in this category have coverage under Section 1931 of the Social Security Act, but some may have coverage under Section 1115 waivers.

The "Other Medicaid Eligibility" category could either be the ACA Medicaid expansion implemented through state plan rules or coverage provided through a Section 1115 waiver.

Individuals with incomes that fall in the "Coverage Gap" category do not have access to full Medicaid coverage or exchange subsidized coverage.

"Subsidized Exchange Coverage Eligibility" is available to individuals with household incomes from 100% FPL through 400% FPL. The ACA provides premium tax credits to individuals with household income between 100% and 400% of FPL who do not have access to minimum essential coverage, and these individuals with income between 100% and 250% FPL could be eligible for cost-sharing subsidies.

FPL: Federal poverty level. In 2014, the federal poverty level (100% of FPL) is $11,670 for an individual and $4,060 for each additional family member in the lower 48 states and the District of Columbia.

Figure A-2. State-by-State Medicaid and Exchange Subsidized Coverage Income Eligibility Levels for Parents with Dependent Children up to 250% of FPL.(As of January 1, 2014).

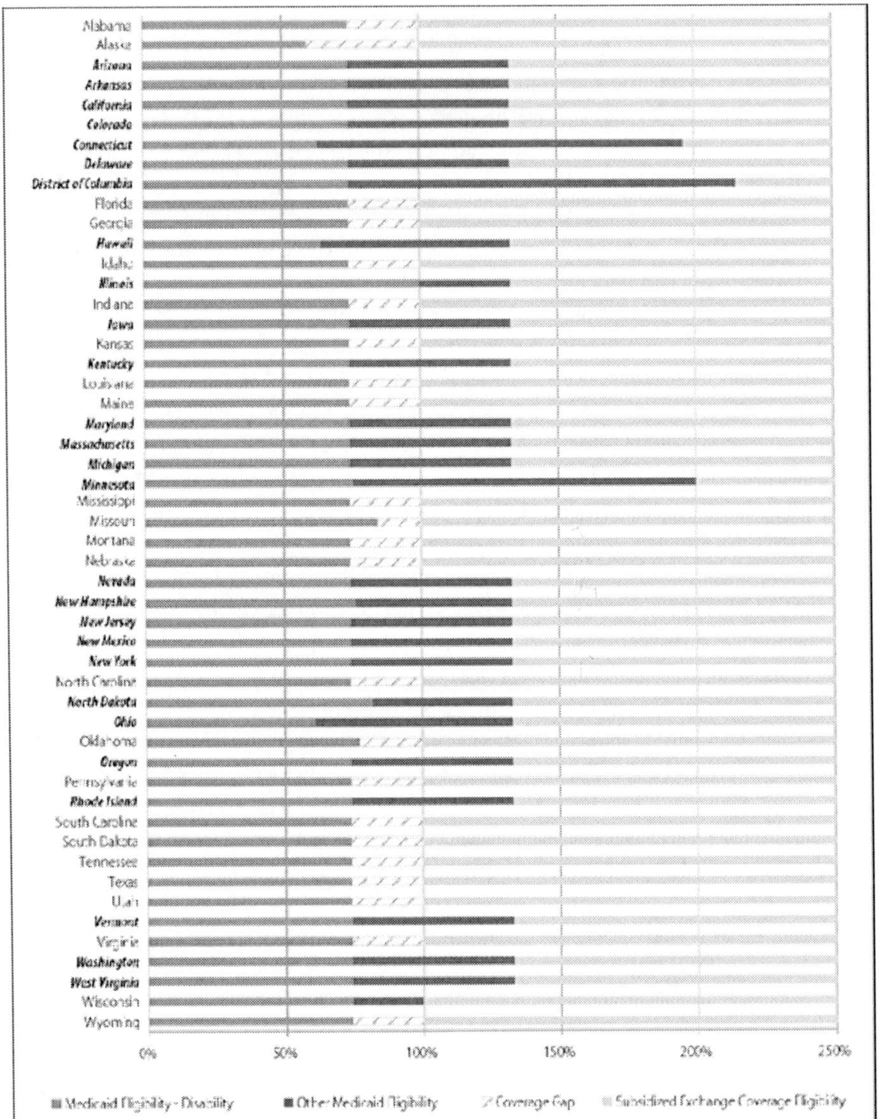

Source: Centers for Medicare & Medicaid Services, "State Medicaid and CHIP Income Eligibility Standards Effective January 1, 2014," October 24, 2013; Medicaid and CHIP Payment and Access Commission, Report to Congress on Medicaid and CHIP, March 2014.

Notes: States in bold are states that have decided to implement the ACA Medicaid expansion. Most states implemented the expansion on January 1, 2014, but Michigan implemented the expansion on April 1, 2014 and New Hampshire plans to implement the ACA Medicaid expansion on July 1, 2014.

The "Medicaid Eligibility – Disability" category is based on states' eligibility levels for SSI recipients in most states and states' 209(b) eligibility level for 209(b) states. In states that have implemented the expansion, an adult with disabilities may have access to different benefit coverage through the ACA Medicaid expansion eligibility pathway (i.e., eligible for Medicaid based solely on their low-income status) than the adults with disabilities that have Medicaid coverage through the SSI eligibility pathway (i.e., eligible for Medicaid based being low-income and disabled).

The "Other Medicaid Eligibility" category could either be the ACA Medicaid expansion implemented through state plan rules or coverage provided through a Section 1115 waiver.

Individuals with incomes that fall in the "Coverage Gap" category do not have access to full Medicaid coverage or exchange subsidized coverage.

"Subsidized Exchange Coverage Eligibility" is available to individuals with household incomes from 100% FPL through 400% FPL. The ACA provides premium tax credits to individuals with household income between 100% and 400% of FPL who do not have access to minimum essential coverage, and these individuals with income between 100% and 250% FPL could be eligible for cost-sharing subsidies.

FPL: Federal poverty level. In 2014, the federal poverty level (100% of FPL) is $11,670 for an individual and $4,060 for each additional family member in the lower 48 states and the District of Columbia.

Figure A-3. State-by-State Medicaid and Exchange Subsidized Coverage Income Eligibility Levels for Adults with Disabilities up to 250% of FPL . (As of January 1, 2014).

APPENDIX B. ESTIMATES OF STATE-BY-STATE IMPACT OF ACA MEDICAID EXPANSION

The potential impact of the ACA Medicaid expansion varies significantly from state to state. In terms of expenditures, while the federal government will be funding a vast majority of the ACA Medicaid expansion, the estimated state share of the ACA Medicaid expansion expenditures range from states that already provide Medicaid coverage to the expansion population saving money to states with the largest coverage gains seeing increases to state Medicaid expenditures. Medicaid enrollment is estimated to increase at varying rates from state to state due to the current variation in states' Medicaid income eligibility levels for parents and childless adults.

Table B-1 shows the estimated state-by-state impact of the ACA Medicaid expansion on Medicaid expenditures and enrollment for 2022 *if* a state chooses to implement the expansion.[80] According to the data in this table from an Urban Institute analysis, if all states chose to implement the ACA Medicaid expansion, Medicaid expenditures for 2022 would be $122.8 billion ($117.4 billion in federal funds and $5.4 billion in state funds) higher than if no states chose to implement the expansion. Also, if all states chose to implement the expansion, Medicaid enrollment would be 15.5 million higher in 2022 than if no states chose to implement the expansion.[81]

Table B-1. State-by-State Estimates of the Impact of the ACA Medicaid Expansion on Medicaid Expenditures and Enrollment, 2022

	Estimated Medicaid Expenditures						Estimated Medicaid Enrollment	
	Medicaid Expenditures for ACA Medicaid Expansion ($ in millions)			Percentage Change in Medicaid Expenditures with ACA Medicaid Expansion			Medicaid Enrollment for ACA Medicaid Expansion (in Millions)	Percent Increase above Medicaid Enrollment without ACA Medicaid Expansion
State	Federal	State	Total	Federal	State	Total		
Alabama	$2,102	$246	$2,348	29.6%	8.0%	23.1%	313	36.1%
Alaska	$213	$31	$244	13.7%	2.4%	8.6%	37	30.1%
Arizona	$1,530	$166	$1,696	14.3%	3.3%	10.8%	238	16.8%
Arkansas	$1,828	$212	$2,041	31.8%	9.3%	25.4%	233	35.0%
California	$10,008	$1,347	$11,356	18.9%	2.7%	11.1%	1,860	18.0%
Colorado	$1,503	$188	$1,691	34.4%	4.7%	20.1%	225	39.0%
Connecticut	$1,196	-$109	$1,086	18.7%	-1.8%	8.8%	150	29.1%
Delaware	$292	-$168	$124	16.4%	-12.5%	4.0%	16	8.3%
District of Columbia	$123	$15	$138	4.7%	1.4%	3.7%	26	16.5%
Florida	$9,645	$1,186	$10,831	46.5%	7.7%	30.1%	1,276	45.2%
Georgia	$4,918	$573	$5,492	41.6%	10.3%	31.6%	698	41.5%
Hawaii	$486	-$36	$451	28.9%	-2.4%	14.2%	62	29.2%
Idaho	$477	$55	$533	20.3%	6.3%	16.5%	88	40.7%
Illinois	$3,160	$455	$3,615	17.5%	2.7%	10.3%	495	21.2%
Indiana	$2,591	$279	$2,870	27.3%	6.3%	20.6%	495	48.8%
Iowa	$572	-$40	$532	11.9%	-1.4%	7.0%	72	15.2%
Kansas	$767	$108	$875	19.6%	4.0%	13.3%	169	45.3%
Kentucky	$2,627	$301	$2,928	30.7%	9.0%	24.6%	268	33.5%
Louisiana	$2,312	$280	$2,592	27.2%	5.4%	18.9%	398	37.9%
Maine	$457	-$70	$387	12.6%	-3.6%	6.9%	45	14.5%
Maryland	$1,749	-$150	$1,598	23.1%	-2.1%	10.7%	146	17.7%
Massachusetts	$1,135	-$1,031	$103	8.1%	-7.8%	0.4%	16	1.1%
Michigan	$2,567	$351	$2,918	16.8%	4.9%	13.0%	345	17.8%

	Estimated Medicaid Expenditures						Estimated Medicaid Enrollment	
	Medicaid Expenditures for ACA Medicaid Expansion ($ in millions)			Percentage Change in Medicaid Expenditures with ACA Medicaid Expansion			Medicaid Enrollment for ACA Medicaid Expansion (in Millions)	Percent Increase above Medicaid Enrollment without ACA Medicaid Expansion
State	Federal	State	Total	Federal	State	Total		
Minnesota	$818	$108	$926	8.2%	1.1%	4.7%	105	13.4%
Mississippi	$2,121	$241	$2,362	32.7%	11.4%	27.4%	231	31.8%
Missouri	$2,590	$336	$2,926	24.6%	5.8%	18.0%	383	37.6%
Montana	$301	$41	$342	19.9%	6.1%	15.7%	64	49.6%
Nebraska	$444	$55	$499	16.6%	2.9%	10.9%	88	37.1%
Nevada	$816	$109	$924	38.4%	7.2%	25.5%	137	48.6%
New Hampshire	$351	$42	$393	19.8%	2.7%	11.8%	42	30.2%
New Jersey	$2,209	$307	$2,516	17.9%	2.7%	10.6%	291	30.1%
New Mexico	$732	$74	$806	14.2%	3.4%	11.0%	208	41.4%
New York	$8,642	-$5,186	$3,456	12.9%	-8.3%	2.7%	320	6.2%
North Carolina	$5,781	$690	$6,471	32.8%	7.6%	24.2%	568	34.4%
North Dakota	$341	$45	$387	30.7%	6.3%	21.1%	32	44.4%
Ohio	$7,809	$920	$8,729	34.4%	7.4%	24.8%	684	32.5%
Oklahoma	$1,252	$154	$1,405	21.1%	4.8%	15.3%	204	29.8%
Oregon	$1,913	$164	$2,077	35.6%	5.7%	25.2%	400	74.8%
Pennsylvania	$5,505	$645	$6,150	23.8%	3.6%	15.0%	542	26.0%
Rhode Island	$429	$55	$484	16.5%	2.5%	10.0%	40	22.0%
South Carolina	$2,312	$265	$2,577	31.9%	9.0%	25.3%	312	35.9%
South Dakota	$307	$36	$343	25.0%	5.0%	17.6%	44	37.9%
Tennessee	$3,328	$390	$3,718	25.5%	6.2%	19.2%	363	26.0%
Texas	$9,582	$1,222	$10,804	29.9%	5.6%	20.1%	1,805	42.1%
Utah	$784	$88	$872	24.7%	7.7%	20.2%	189	57.1%
Vermont	$156	-$135	$22	9.5%	-12.5%	0.8%	3	2.0%
Virginia	$2,144	$285	$2,429	29.8%	4.2%	17.3%	327	38.5%
Washington	$1,221	$77	$1,298	14.6%	1.0%	7.9%	137	11.7%
West Virginia	$1,278	$144	$1,423	28.3%	9.2%	23.3%	116	30.9%
Wisconsin	$1,753	$56	$1,808	20.0%	1.0%	12.6%	211	23.3%
Wyoming	$198	$26	$223	23.5%	3.9%	14.8%	27	34.2%
National Total	$117,375	$5,443	$122,819	23.0%	1.5%	14.0%	15,544	26.8%

Source: John Holahan, Matthew Buettgens, and Caitlin Carroll, et al., The Costs and Coverage Implications of the ACA Medicaid Expansion: National and State-by-State Analysis, Kaiser Commission on Medicaid and the Uninsured, Publication #8384, November 2012, Tables 8 and 9.

Notes: The state-by-state analysis was conducted using the Urban Institute's Health Insurance Policy Simulation Model (HIPSM), which is a detailed microsimulation model of the health care system that estimates the cost and coverage effects of proposed health care policy options.

End Notes

[1] For more information about the Medicaid program, see CRS Report R43357, Medicaid: An Overview, coordinated by Alison Mitchell.

[2] For an overview of Medicaid financing issues, see CRS Report R42640, Medicaid Financing and Expenditures, by Alison Mitchell.

[3] For more information about the FMAP rate, see CRS Report R42941, Medicaid's Federal Medical Assistance Percentage (FMAP), FY2014, by Alison Mitchell and Evelyne P. Baumrucker.

[4] Most legal permanent residents that have been in the United States for more than five years can be eligible for Medicaid if they meet the other eligibility requirements, while most legal permanent residents during their first five years, undocumented immigrants, and immigrants in the United States on a temporary basis are generally ineligible for Medicaid.

[5] Section 1115 of the Social Security Act gives the Secretary of Health and Human Services authority to approve experimental, pilot, or demonstration projects that promote the objectives of the Medicaid program.

[6] Not all individuals eligible for Medicaid have Medicaid coverage because individuals may not know they are eligible or they may choose to not enroll in the program. (Kaiser Commission on Medicaid the Uninsured, The Coverage Gap: Uninsured Poor Adults in States that Do Not Expand Medicaid, October 2013.)

[7] The ACA also requires states to provide Medicaid coverage to certain individuals who age out of foster care, up to age 26 regardless of their income, and do not qualify under one of the other mandatory groups noted above starting in 2014. In addition, the ACA increased the federally mandated Medicaid eligibility level for children ages six through 18 from 100% to 133% of FPL beginning in 2014.

[8] On November 21, 2011, President Obama signed into law P.L. 112-56, which changes the definition of income to include non-taxable Social Security in the definition of MAGI. For more information about MAGI, see CRS Report R41997, Definition of Income for Certain Medicaid Provisions and Premium Credits in ACA, coordinated by Christine Scott.

[9] The ACA provided states with the option to implement the ACA Medicaid expansion earlier than 2014. During the transitional period between April 1, 2010, and January 1, 2014, states had the option to expand Medicaid to individuals eligible under the new eligibility group up to 133% of FPL as long as the state did not extend coverage to (1) individuals with higher income before those with lower income or (2) parents unless their children are enrolled in the state plan, a waiver, or in other health coverage. Eight states (California, Colorado, Connecticut, Illinois, Minnesota, New Jersey, Ohio, and Washington) and the District of Columbia elected to implement the ACA Medicaid expansion prior to 2014.

[10] For more information about the Supreme Court decision, see CRS Report R42367, Medicaid and Federal Grant Conditions After NFIB v. Sebelius: Constitutional Issues and Analysis, by Kenneth R. Thomas.

[11] As with making any other change to a state's Medicaid state plan, in order to end the ACA Medicaid expansion, states would be required to submit a state plan amendment to CMS for approval. (Centers for Medicare & Medicaid Services, Frequently Asked Questions on Exchanges, Market Reforms and Medicaid, December 2012.)

[12] Enrollment to new enrollees was closed in Arizona and Colorado.

[13] As of January 2013, the following 18 states provide Medicaid coverage with limited benefits to adults without dependent children: Arkansas, California, Idaho, Indiana (enrollment closed), Iowa, Maine (enrollment closed), Maryland, Massachusetts, Michigan (enrollment closed),

Minnesota, New Jersey, New Mexico (enrollment closed), Oklahoma, Oregon (enrollment closed), Utah (enrollment closed to non-working childless adults), Vermont, Washington (enrollment closed), and Wisconsin (enrollment closed).

[14] Medicaid and CHIP Payment and Access Commission, Report to Congress on Medicaid and CHIP, March 2013, Table 110 on page 94.

[15] AFDC was a federal entitlement program to low-income families with children that provided cash assistance, which was replaced with Temporary Assistance for Needy Families (TANF), signed into law in 1996 as part of the Personal Responsibility and Work Opportunity Reconciliation Act (PRWORA, P.L. 104-193). Under AFDC, those receiving AFDC benefits were guaranteed Medicaid eligibility, but TANF and Medicaid eligibility are not linked. PRWORA established a new eligibility category for these low-income families under Section 1931 of the Social Security Act, which requires states to cover parents who meet the AFDC eligibility criteria in place on July 16, 1996. The AFDC eligibility criteria had a categorical and a financial requirement. The categorical requirement is that the individual is a single parent or a two-parent family in which the principal earner is unemployed. The financial requirement is the AFDC income eligibility levels in place on July 16, 1996, which vary by state.

[16] States are required to continue Medicaid benefits for certain low-income families who would otherwise lose coverage because of changes in their income. This continuation of benefits is known as transitional medical assistance (TMA). Federal law permanently requires four months of TMA for families who lose Medicaid eligibility, and currently, Section 1925 of the Social Security Act requires states to provide at least 6 and up to 12 months of coverage through TMA. Section 1925 of TMA relies on regular extensions of its authority and funding by Congress.

[17] The following 12 states have Medicaid eligibility thresholds for full Medicaid coverage for parents with dependent children at or above 133% or FPL: Connecticut, District of Columbia, Hawaii, Illinois, Maine, Massachusetts, Minnesota, New Jersey, New York, Rhode Island, Vermont, and Wisconsin.

[18] The following 13 states provide limited Medicaid coverage to parents with dependent children: Arkansas, California, Idaho, Indiana, Iowa, Massachusetts, Minnesota, New Mexico (enrollment closed), Oklahoma, Oregon (enrollment closed), Utah (enrollment closed to non-working childless adults), Vermont, and Washington (enrollment closed).

[19] Medicaid and CHIP Payment and Access Commission, Report to Congress on Medicaid and CHIP, March 2013, Table 110 on page 94.

[20] In 2014, the maximum federal SSI payment, referred to as the federal benefit rate, is $721 per month for an individual living independently and $1,082 for a couple living independently in 2014, which translates to 74% of the FPL in 2014. For more information about SSI income and resource limits, see CRS Report RS20294, Supplemental Security Income (SSI): Income/Resource Limits and Accounts Exempt from Benefit Determinations, by William R. Morton.

[21] There are 11 209(b) states: Connecticut, Hawaii, Illinois, Indiana, Minnesota, Missouri, New Hampshire, North Dakota, Ohio, Oklahoma, and Virginia.

[22] For more information about the optional Medicaid eligibility pathways for nonelderly, disabled adults, see CRS Report R41899, Medicaid Eligibility for Persons Age 65+ and Individuals with Disabilities: 2009 State Profiles, by Kirsten J. Colello and Scott R. Talaga.

[23] The MAGI income counting rules also apply to most other Medicaid eligibility groups.

[24] While the Internal Revenue Service's definition of MAGI excludes non-taxable social security benefits, P.L. 112-56, enacted on November 21, 2011, changed the definition of income for Medicaid eligibility to include such non-taxable social security benefits.

[25] For more information about MAGI rules, see CRS Report R41997, Definition of Income for Certain Medicaid Provisions and Premium Credits in ACA, coordinated by Christine Scott.

[26] The traditional Medicaid program covers a wide variety of mandatory services (e.g., inpatient hospital services, lab/x-ray services, physician care, nursing facility care for persons aged 21 and over), and other services at state option (e.g., prescribed drugs, physician-directed clinic services, physical therapy, prosthetic devices) to the majority of Medicaid beneficiaries across the United States. Within broad federal guidelines, states define the amount, duration, and scope of these benefits. Thus, even mandatory services are not identical from state to state.

[27] For more information about ABPs, see CRS Report R43357, Medicaid: An Overview, coordinated by Alison Mitchell.

[28] For more information about coverage of long-term services and supports under ABPs, see CRS Report R43328, Medicaid Coverage of Long-Term Services and Supports, by Kirsten J. Colello.

[29] Department of Health and Human Services, "Medicaid and Children's Health Insurance Programs: Essential Health Benefits in Alternative Benefit Plans, Eligibility Notices, Fair Hearing and Appeal Processes, and Premiums and Cost Sharing; Exchanges: Eligibility and Enrollment," 78 Federal Register 42160, July 15, 2013.

[30] Generally determined annually, the FMAP formula is designed so that the federal government pays a larger portion of Medicaid costs in states with lower per capita incomes relative to the national average (and vice versa for states with higher per capita incomes). FMAP rates have a statutory minimum of 50% and a statutory maximum of 83%. For FY2014, regular FMAP rates range from 50.00% to 73.05%. For more information about the FMAP rate, see CRS Report R42941, Medicaid's Federal Medical Assistance Percentage (FMAP), FY2014, by Alison Mitchell and Evelyne P. Baumrucker.

[31] The coverage must include inpatient hospital services and cannot consist only of the following: premium assistance (or Medicaid coverage otherwise dependent on employer coverage or contribution), hospital-only plans, high-deductible health plans, or Health Opportunity Accounts under Section 1938 of the Social Security Act.

[32] A state that offered health benefits coverage to only parents or only nonpregnant childless adults is not considered to be an expansion state; both groups must have been covered as specified for a state to be classified as an expansion state.

[33] Communication with the Centers for Medicare & Medicaid Services March 4, 2014.

[34] Pennsylvania is the only state that meets the definition of an "expansion state" that has not implemented the ACA Medicaid expansion, which means Pennsylvania is not currently receiving the "expansion state" FMAP rate.

[35] Expansion state FMAP formula = [regular FMAP + (newly eligible FMAP – regular FMAP) * transition percentage equal to 50% in CY2014, 60% in CY2015, 70% in CY2016, 80% in CY2017, 90% in CY2018, and 100% in CY2019+].

[36] Centers for Medicare & Medicaid Services, Frequently Asked Questions on Exchanges, Market Reforms and Medicaid, December 10, 2012.

[37] Under an approved Section 1115 waiver, states may have limited authority to make Medicaid disproportionate share hospital (DSH) payments under Section 1923 of the Social Security Act because all or a portion of their DSH allotment is included in the budget neutrality calculation for an expansion of Medicaid eligibility under an approved Section 1115 waiver

or to fund uncompensated care pools and/or safety net care pools. For more information about Medicaid DSH payments, see CRS Report R42865, Medicaid Disproportionate Share Hospital Payments, by Alison Mitchell.

[38] Congressional Budget Office, The Budget and Economic Outlook: 2014 to 2024, February 2014.

[39] Ibid.

[40] Genevieve M. Kenney, Lisa Dubay, Stephen Zuckerman, and Michael Huntress, Opting Out of the Medicaid Expansion under the ACA: How Many Uninsured Adults Would not Be Eligible for Medicaid?, The Urban Institute Health Policy Center, July 5, 2012; Benjamin D. Sommers and Arnold M. Epstein, "Perspective: Why States Are So Miffed about Medicaid - Economics, Politics, and the "Woodwork Effect"," The New England Journal of Medicine, vol. 365, no. 2, pp. 100-102 (July 14, 2011).

[41] Congressional Budget Office, Updated Estimates of the Insurance Coverage Provisions of the Affordable Care Act, April 2014.

[42] Ibid.

[43] Neither CMS nor CBO provide state level estimates of these changes. The appendix provides estimates conducted by the Urban Institute.

[44] Adrianne Appel, "New Hampshire: Gov. Hassan Signs Bill to Expand Medicaid Coverage Via Waiver Plan," Bloomberg BNA, March 31, 2014.

[45] States' decisions are based on CRS's monitoring of state activity through media outlets and state tracking of decisions done by CMS, State Refor(u)m, the Kaiser Family Foundation, the Advisory Board Company, and Avalere.

[46] U.S. Census Bureau, American Community Survey, 2012; Medicaid and CHIP Payment and Access Commission, Report to the Congress on Medicaid and CHIP, March 2013.

[47] For more information about how states make the decision whether or not to implement the ACA Medicaid expansion, see CRS Report WSLG433, Who Gets to Say Yes or No to the Medicaid Expansion - The Governor or the State Legislature?, by Kathleen S. Swendiman.

[48] Jason Kane, "'Private option' Medicaid expansion to continue in Arkansas," PBS Newshour, March 5, 2014.

[49] Norma Love, "New Hampshire Medicaid expansion goes to governor," boston.com, March 25, 2014; Adrianne Appel, "New Hampshire: Gov. Hassan Signs Bill to Expand Medicaid Coverage Via Waiver Plan," Bloomberg BNA, March 31, 2014.

[50] Kirsten Stewart and Robert Gehrke, "Utah guv: Medicaid will expand," The Salt Lake Tribune, January 23, 2014.

[51] Associated Press, "General Assembly returns for special session," The Washington Post, March 23, 2014.

[52] State Refor(u)m, Governors Address Medicaid Expansion in "State of the State" Speeches, March 2013.

[53] Under premium assistance, states are permitted to use federal Medicaid funds to subsidize the cost of private health insurance coverage for Medicaid enrollees in lieu of direct Medicaid coverage.

[54] Health savings accounts are accounts with funding available to cover the cost of health care services.

[55] Julie Plotrowski, "Health Policy Brief: Premium Assistance in Medicaid," Health Affairs, June 6, 2013.

[56] CRS Report R42663, Health Insurance Exchanges Under the Patient Protection and Affordable Care Act (ACA), by Bernadette Fernandez and Annie L. Mach.

[57] Arkansas Health Care Independence Program (Private Option), CMS Special Terms and Conditions (September 27, 13), available at http://www.medicaid.gov/Medicaid-CHIP-Program-Information/By-Topics/Waivers/1115/downloads/ ar/ar-private-option-ca.pdf.

[58] Iowa Market Place Choice Plan, CMS Special Terms and Conditions (December 30, 2013), available at http://www.medicaid.gov/Medicaid-CHIP-Program-Information/By-Topics/Waivers/1115/downloads/ia/iamarketplace-choice-plan-ca.pdf.

[59] Adrianne Appel, "New Hampshire: Gov. Hassan Signs Bill to Expand Medicaid Coverage Via Waiver Plan," Bloomberg BNA, March 31, 2014.

[60] Elana Gordan, "What's Next For Pennsylvania's Medicaid Expansion?," Kaiser Health News, March 10, 2014.

[61] Phil Galewitz, "Arkansas' Medicaid Experiment, Key to Obamacare Expansion, On Ropes," Kaiser Health News, February 10, 2014.

[62] Medicaid and CHIP Payment and Access Commission, Report to the Congress on Medicaid and CHIP, March 2014.

[63] Centers for Medicare & Medicaid Services, Medicaid and the Affordable Care Act: Premium Assistance, March 2013.

[64] The ACA allows a state to apply to the Secretary of HHS for a waiver of specific requirements with respect to health insurance coverage within that state for plan years beginning on or after January 1, 2017. The state may apply to waive any or all of the following: requirements relating to establishment of qualified health plans; requirement for the state to have an exchange; requirement to offer premium tax credits and cost-sharing reductions through an exchange; requirement for individuals to maintain coverage (individual mandate); and the penalties imposed on employers whose employees receive premium tax credits.

[65] Centers for Medicare & Medicaid Services, Medicaid and the Affordable Care Act: Premium Assistance, March 2013.

[66] Alexandra Gates, Robin Rudowitz, and MaryBeth Musumeci, Medicaid Expansion in Michigan, The Kaiser Commission on Medicaid and the Uninsured, January 17, 2014.

[67] Communication with the Michigan Department of Community Health on May 12, 2014.

[68] Reid Wilson, "Republicans seek political cover to accept Medicaid expansion money," The Washington Post, February 25, 2014.

[69] Alexandra Gates, Robin Rudowitz, and Samantha Artiga, Healthy Indiana Plan and the Affordable Care Act, Kaiser Commission on Medicaid and the Uninsured, December 2013.

[70] The definition of minimum essential coverage is broad. It includes Medicare Part A, Medicaid, the State Children's Health Insurance Program (CHIP), Tricare, the TRICARE for Life program, the veteran's health care program, the Peace Corps program, a government plan (local, state, federal) including the Federal Employees Health Benefits Program (FEHBP) and any plan established by an Indian tribal government, any plan offered in the individual, small group or large group market, a grandfathered health plan, and any other health benefits coverage, such as a state health benefits risk pool, as recognized by the Secretary of HHS in coordination with the Treasury Secretary.

[71] In general, legal permanent residents within their first five years in the country are not eligible for Medicaid, so the ACA extended premium tax credits to these individuals with income below 400% of FPL so that they would be able to purchase health insurance through the exchanges. After five years, legal permanent residents are eligible for Medicaid according to the Medicaid eligibility levels in their state. For more information about noncitizen eligibility for Medicaid, see CRS Report RL33809, Noncitizen Eligibility for Federal Public Assistance: Policy Overview and Trends, by Ruth Ellen Wasem.

[72] Centers for Medicare & Medicaid Services, Frequently Asked Questions on Exchanges, Market Reforms and Medicaid, December 2012.

[73] Kaiser Commission on Medicaid and the Uninsured, The Coverage Gap: Uninsured Poor Adults in States that Do Not Expand Medicaid, October 2013.

[74] The employer penalty was supposed to go into effect in 2014, but on July 2, 2013, the Obama Administration announced that it is delaying, until 2015, the enforcement and associated reporting requirements related to the employer penalty. For more information about the delay to the employer penalty, see CRS Report R43150, Delay in Implementation of Potential Employer Penalties Under ACA, by Bernadette Fernandez and Annie L. Mach.

[75] A "large employer" is defined in the ACA (as related to the employer penalty) as an employer who employed an average of at least 50 full-time equivalent employees (FTEs) on business days during the preceding calendar year.

[76] For more information about the employer penalty, see CRS Report R41159, Potential Employer Penalties Under the Patient Protection and Affordable Care Act (ACA), by Julie M. Whittaker.

[77] For more information about Medicaid DSH payments, see CRS Report R42865, Medicaid Disproportionate Share Hospital Payments, by Alison Mitchell.

[78] Toluse Olorunnipa, "Obamacare Cutbacks Shut Hospitals Where Medicaid Went Unexpanded," Bloomberg Government, November 25, 2013. Letter from the Republican Governors Public Policy Committee to President Barack Obama dated July 10, 2012, available at http://www.scribd.com/doc/99730375/Medicaid-and-Exchange-Letter-Final. Sarah Kliff, "The super wonky reason states may join the Medicaid expansion," The Washington Post, July 8, 2012. Bob Neal, The Fiscal and Economic Impacts of Medicaid Expansion in Mississippi, 2014-2025, Mississippi Public Universities University Research Center, October 2012.

[79] Special benefit rules apply for the Medically Needy pathway.

[80] Neither CMS nor CBO provide state level estimates of the impact of the ACA Medicaid expansion on Medicaid expenditures and enrollment. As a result, this table uses state level estimates conducted by the Urban Institute.

[81] John Holahan, Matthew Buettgens, and Caitlin Carroll, et al., The Costs and Coverage Implications of the ACA Medicaid Expansion: National and State-by-State Analysis, Kaiser Commission on Medicaid and the Uninsured, Publication #8384, November 2012, Tables 8 and 9.

In: Medicaid Expansion …
Editor: Gail Norman

ISBN: 978-1-63463-442-7

Chapter 2

THE CONSTITUTIONALITY OF FEDERAL GRANT CONDITIONS AFTER *NATIONAL FEDERATION OF INDEPENDENT BUSINESS V. SEBELIUS*[*]

Kenneth R. Thomas

SUMMARY

In March 2010, Congress passed the Patient Protection and Affordable Care Act (ACA). The ACA, among other things, requires states to expand Medicaid eligibility or lose Medicaid funding. Following the enactment of the ACA, state attorneys general and others brought several lawsuits challenging various provisions of the act on constitutional grounds. In *National Federation of Independent Business (NFIB) v. Sebelius,* the Supreme Court, among other things, decided that the enforcement mechanism for the ACA Medicaid expansion, withdrawal of all Medicaid funds, was a violation of the Tenth Amendment. The Court went on to hold, however, that the remedy was to sever that enforcement mechanism, effectively making state participation in the Medicaid expansion voluntary.

---

[*] This is an edited, reformatted and augmented version of a Congressional Research Service publication R42367, prepared for Members and Committees of Congress, dated July 17, 2012.

In the 1987 case of *South Dakota v. Dole,* the Supreme Court held that, in order for a federal grant condition imposed on a state to pass constitutional muster under the Spending Clause, the condition must be related to the particular national projects or programs to which the money was being directed. In addition, in order to comply with the limits of the Tenth Amendment, the level of funds withheld for failure to comply with that condition cannot be coercive. In a controlling opinion in *NFIB*, Justice Roberts suggested that this analysis may vary based on the type of grant condition that was at issue. It is unclear, however, whether *NFIB* significantly changed the *Dole* analysis, or whether the combination of factors that led the Court's decision to limit how ACA Medicaid expansion would be enforced is likely to be repeated.

For instance, if a grant condition is directly related to the expenditure of federal funds in a state program or activity, then, according to Justice Robert's opinion in *NFIB*, the condition is usually constitutional under the Spending Clause. Or even if a grant condition is only generally related to the policy goals of the underlying grant, *NFIB* suggests that withdrawal of all program funds would still, in most foreseeable cases, be constitutional under the Spending Clause and the Tenth Amendment. If a grant condition is unrelated to the general policy goals of the underlying grant, however, then it is most likely unconstitutional under the Spending Clause. This latter standard, however, has been in place since the *Dole* case, and no court has ever struck down a federal law on this basis.

Justice Roberts' concern in *NFIB* arguably dealt with a different question: whether a grant condition attached to a new and independent program (here, the Medicaid expansion) which threatens the funding of an existing program (here Medicaid) is constitutional. In such cases, if the withholding of federal funding represents a significant portion of a state's budget, and there are distinguishing factors among the programs, then that condition may be unconstitutionally coercive under the Tenth Amendment. Justice Roberts did not identify a standard to determine what level of withholding funds would be coercive, or specify what kind of distinguishing factors were necessary. He did conclude, however, that withdrawal of federal program funds which made up ten percent of an average state's budget represented a "gun to the head" and was a form of "economic dragooning."

How courts are to consider grant withdrawals below ten percent, however, is not addressed by the Roberts' opinion, and Justice Roberts declined to speculate where such a line would be drawn. It should be noted, however, that few federal programs even approach the level of Medicaid funds provided to the states. Thus, if the ten percent threshold and the need for distinguishing factors mark the outer limits of Congress's power, then the case may have minimal effect on existing or future federal grant conditions.

BACKGROUND

In March 2010, the 111th Congress passed the Patient Protection and Affordable Care Act[1] as amended by the Health Care and Education Reconciliation Act of 2010.[2] Jointly referred to as the Affordable Care Act (ACA), the ACA expands Medicaid eligibility, increases access to health insurance coverage, expands federal private health insurance market requirements, requires the creation of health insurance exchanges to provide individuals and small employers with access to insurance, and in some instances, mandates the provision and purchasing of health insurance.[3]

Following the enactment of the ACA, state attorneys general and others brought several lawsuits challenging various provisions of the ACA on constitutional grounds.[4] One of these cases included a federalism challenge to the ACA's expansion of Medicaid eligibility. This case, *National Federation of Independent Business (NFIB) v. Sebelius*,[5] addressed the issue of whether withholding Medicaid reimbursement to a state unless that state complies with the expansion of its Medicaid program exceeds Congress's enumerated powers under the Spending Clause and violates the Tenth Amendment. In *NFIB*, the Court held that the withdrawal of all Medicaid funds from the states for failure to comply with the expansion of the program did violate the Tenth Amendment, but that withholding of just the funds associated with that expansion raised no significant constitutional concerns.

Medicaid is an entitlement program that finances the delivery of certain health care services to a specific population. Medicaid is financed jointly by the federal and state governments, and states choose whether or not to participate. Currently all 50 states participate. If a state chooses to participate, it must follow federal rules in order to receive federal reimbursement that offsets most of the state's Medicaid costs. It should be noted, however, that a number of these requirements may be waived, with approval from the Secretary of Health and Human Services (HHS).[6]

In general, Medicaid expansion under the ACA: (1) increases Medicaid eligibility by raising the income criteria for certain people; (2) adds both mandatory and optional benefits to Medicaid; (3) increases the federal matching payments for certain groups of beneficiaries and for particular services provided; (4) provides new requirements and incentives for states to improve quality of care and to encourage more use of preventive services; and (5) makes a number of other Medicaid program changes.[7]

The most significant of these changes amends a section of federal law outlining what states must offer in their Medicaid coverage plans.[8] Starting in

2014, states were to be required to cover adults under age 65 (who are not pregnant and not already covered) with incomes up to 133 percent of the federal poverty level ("FPL").[9] This is a significant change because previously the Medicaid Act did not set a baseline income level for mandatory eligibility. Thus, many states currently do not provide Medicaid to childless adults and cover parents only at much lower income levels.[10] Failure to comply with such expansion could, in theory, result in the withholding of all Medicaid reimbursements to the states, including payments for persons previously covered by the Medicaid program.

The federal government predicted that if all states chose to participate in the Medicaid expansion, enrollment would increase by approximately 16 million by the end of the decade.[11] To finance the expansion, the federal government calculated that its share of Medicaid spending would increase by $434 billion by 2020, and state spending would increase by at least $20 billion over the same time frame.[12] Other estimates suggest that both federal and state costs could be higher.[13]

The constitutional challenge to the Medicaid expansion in *NFIB* was that, under the Spending Clause and the Tenth Amendment, states would be coerced into paying for the increased Medicaid requirements, as the failure to comply with these increased Medicaid requirements might result in the federal government withholding all Medicaid funding. The argument was bolstered by the states noting that Medicaid represents 40 percent of all federal funds that states receive; that the majority of states receive more than $1 billion in Medicaid funding each year; and that this number is projected to increase under the ACA. The states argued that the withdrawal of this aid would have a dramatic effect on the ability of the states to provide health care to their populations,[14] and that the states had no choice but to comply with the Medicaid expansion provisions.

The Spending Clause

The authority of Congress to specify under what conditions the states will receive Medicaid funds is generally considered to be the Spending Clause.[15] Under the Spending Clause, Congress can allocate money to states, private entities, or individuals, but then require those recipients to engage in or refrain from certain activities as a condition of receiving and spending that money. The question arises, however, whether under precepts of federalism, there are limitations on Congress' ability to apply such requirements to the states.

The lines of authority between states and the federal government are, to a significant extent, defined by the United States Constitution and relevant case law regarding federalism. In recent years, the Supreme Court has decided a number of cases that would seem to be a reevaluation of this historical relationship. In particular, a number of these cases have cited the Commerce Clause,[16] the Tenth Amendment,[17] and the Eleventh Amendment of the Constitution as establishing limitations on the power of the federal government over the states.[18]

In contrast to this trend, the Court has generally interpreted congressional power under the Spending Clause expansively, even when that legislation arguably intrudes on state sovereignty. For instance, many areas of federal law that regulate states, such as civil rights statutes,[19] have been enacted pursuant to the Spending Clause. In many situations, such as where these statutes apply to state agencies or institutions, Congress is using its spending power to accomplish goals that cannot be legislated directly because such direct legislation would be unconstitutionally intrusive on state sovereignty or beyond the authority of Congress.[20]

The Tenth Amendment

One of the limits on federal power that would appear to most often stand in contrast with this Spending Clause doctrine is the Tenth Amendment. The Tenth Amendment provides that "powers not delegated to the United States by the Constitution, nor prohibited by it to the States, are reserved to the States respectively, or to the people." The significance of this language has varied over time. For awhile, the Supreme Court interpreted the Tenth Amendment to provide that certain "core" state powers or "functions" would be beyond the authority of the federal government to regulate.[21] The Court, however, soon overruled that decision, suggesting that the states should look for relief from direct federal regulation of state activities through the political process, not through the courts.[22]

Modern Tenth Amendment doctrine may be traced to the Court's 1992 decision in *New York v. United States*.[23] In *New York*, Congress had attempted to regulate in the area of low-level radioactive waste by providing that states must either develop legislation on how to dispose of all low-level radioactive waste generated within the states, or the states would be forced to take title to such waste, which would mean that it became the states' responsibility.[24] The Court found that although Congress had the authority under the Commerce

Clause to regulate low-level radioactive waste, it only had the power to regulate the waste directly. Here, Congress had attempted to require the states to perform the regulation, and decreed that the failure to do so would require the states to deal with the financial consequences of owning large quantities of radioactive waste. In effect, Congress sought to "commandeer" the legislative process of the states.[25] In the *New York* case, the Court found that this power was not found in the text or structure of the Constitution, and it was thus a violation of the Tenth Amendment.

A later case presented the question of the extent to which Congress could regulate through a state's executive branch officers. *Printz v. United States,*[26] which involved the Brady Handgun Act, required state and local law enforcement officers to conduct background checks on prospective handgun purchasers within five business days of an attempted purchase.[27] This portion of the act was challenged under the Tenth Amendment, under the theory that Congress was without authority to "commandeer" state executive branch officials. After a historical study of federal commandeering of state officials, the Court concluded that commandeering of state executive branch officials was, like commandeering of the legislature, outside of Congress's power, and consequently a violation of the Tenth Amendment.[28]

In the instant case, if the federal government had directly required states to fund and implement new responsibilities under the Medicaid expansion, then it would appear likely that a legal challenge could be made that Congress was commandeering the states to implement a federal program. However, while Congress will be requiring states to provide expanded service under Medicaid as a condition of receiving federal funds under that program, there is no requirement on states to accept those funds. For this reason, a challenge to the Medicaid expansion does not fit comfortably into the commandeering line of cases. Since the state is free to choose not to receive such funds, then it is difficult to argue that such state is being directly commandeered, as was the case in *New York* and *Printz*.

However, in a separate line of cases, the Supreme Court has considered the question of whether conditioning a government benefit on the waiver of a constitutionally based right may in itself be a constitutional violation. The legal theory behind these cases is generally referred to (although not always explicitly by the courts) as the doctrine of "unconstitutional conditions." Thus, the question which was before the Supreme Court in *NFIB* was whether a state may constitutionally be required to accede to the Medicaid expansion as a condition of receiving federal funds, despite the fact that, under *New York* and *Printz*, such requirements could not be imposed directly.

Voluntary Waiver of States' Rights

The Supreme Court has long held that constitutional rights may be "waived" voluntarily by either individuals, private entities, or states. Even rights of the most profound importance, such as the right of the individual to challenge the imposition of capital punishment under the Eighth Amendment, may knowingly be waived.[29] A more difficult question arises, however, where some form of inducement is offered that is conditioned on such a waiver, bringing into question whether such waiver is voluntary.

In some cases, such a waiver is considered unremarkable, even though the rights waived are significant and the inducements are serious. For example, the Court has held that as a result of plea bargaining, a criminal defendant may choose to waive his or her right to a trial in exchange for a reduction in the level of penalty to which the defendant may be subjected.[30] Arguably, such an inducement is unlikely to violate a defendant's rights because the defendant can use his or her estimation of the likelihood of conviction in deciding whether to accept such a bargain.

In other cases, it may be more difficult to evaluate whether the circumstances surrounding the waiver of a constitutional right are so coercive as to in some way infringe on the waived right. In other words, in some cases a grant requirement may be an "unconstitutional condition," because the recipient of the grant is being asked to give up a constitutional right to receive the federal benefit. It is of some concern that the Court has not laid out a universal doctrine for evaluating which rights may be made as a condition of receiving a government benefit, and what circumstances must be in place for such conditioning to be valid. Rather, the Court appears to vary significantly in its approach, changing its level of scrutiny based on the nature of the governmental inducements and the importance of the constitutional right which is sought to be waived. At least one scholar has suggested that attempting to discern doctrinal consistencies in the area yields little predictive benefit.[31]

Despite this lack of a universal approach, there are two consistent themes in evaluating the possibility that a required waiver of a constitutional right is an "unconstitutional condition." First, a court will evaluate whether there is a logical relationship between the purposes of the overall legislation and the burden imposed (relatedness).[32] In addition, a court will evaluate the subjective value of the governmental interest to determine whether the threatened loss of the benefit so outweighs the burdens of compliance that the recipient has little choice but to comply (coercion).[33] The relative weight of two of these factors and their relationship to each other, however, may vary depending on the circumstance to which they are applied.

It should be noted that many recipients of federal money are private individuals or entities. In general, the Court has been more sensitive to grant conditions that limit these private grant recipients' constitutional rights than it has been to states. One theory suggests that the reason for this deference is that the Supreme Court is most concerned in the area of unconstitutional conditions when there is an imbalance in bargaining power, such as can occur between individuals and the government. Such imbalances are particularly exacerbated when the government holds a monopoly power over the offered benefit.[34] For this reason, the doctrine of unconstitutional conditions has been most robust when the cases have involved private individuals being limited in the exercise of either personal autonomy or property rights.[35]

Prior to *NFIB*, the doctrine of unconstitutional conditions had not been successfully invoked by the states. For instance, neither the Supreme Court nor any other court had held that a grant condition imposed on a state failed either a relatedness or coercion test.[36] In part, this appears to reflect the view that states, holding far more financial and political power than most private entities, were more able to withstand federal coercion. Consequently, the Supreme Court's decision in *NFIB*, to the extent that it represents a shift in the Court's approach to Spending Clause cases, could have a significant impact on federal authority to impose spending conditions on states.

An example of a grant condition that does not violate the Tenth Amendment can be found in *South Dakota v. Dole.*[37] In *Dole*, the Court found that Congress was well within its authority to withhold five percent of federal highway funds from states in which the age for purchase of alcohol was below twenty-one years.[38] In that case, the State of South Dakota, which permitted nineteen-year-olds to purchase beer, brought suit challenging the grant requirement, arguing that the law was an invalid exercise of Congress's power under the Spending Clause[39] to provide for the "general welfare." Finding that the legislation was a clear exercise of Congress's power under the Spending Clause,[40] the Court went on to hold that, under this Clause, the condition must be related to the particular national projects or programs to which the money was being directed (relatedness).[41] Further, the Court considered whether other constitutional provisions, such as the Tenth Amendment, may independently bar the conditional grant of federal funds.[42]

The relatedness requirement was of some concern to the Court. In *Dole*, however, the congressional condition imposing a specific drinking age was found to be related to the national concern of safe interstate travel, which was one of the main purposes for expenditure of highway funds.[43] It should be noted that this standard of relatedness was relatively lenient, in that the condition was only indirectly related to how the federal money was being spent or to the specific federal projects involved. Instead, the condition was related to the overall regulatory goal (transportation safety) of the provided funds.

Next, the Court turned to the question of whether the Tenth Amendment (which provides that state legislatures or executive branch officials may not be "commandeered") was an independent constitutional bar to the grant condition. The argument that the Court considered was whether the grant condition was intruding on the state's authority to regulate alcohol or on the right of the state legislature to be free from federal directives as to how to legislate regarding its own state liquor laws. The Court held that because the state had voluntarily agreed to comply with the grant condition in question, the statute was not a violation of the Tenth Amendment.

The Court did suggest, however, that there were some Tenth Amendment limits to Congress's power under the Spending Clause, noting that financial inducements offered by Congress might be so coercive as to pass the point at which "pressure turns into compulsion."[44] In *Dole*, however, the percentage of highway funds that were to be withheld from a state with a drinking age below twenty-one was relatively small, so that Congress's program did not coerce the state to enact higher minimum drinking ages than it would otherwise choose.

NFIB v. Sebelius

In *NFIB*, the Supreme Court reviewed a decision by the U.S. Court of Appeals for the Eleventh Circuit (Eleventh Circuit) regarding a challenge to the Medicaid expansion.[45] In its opinion, the Eleventh Circuit considered a Spending Clause/Tenth Amendment "coercion" challenge to the Medicaid expansion provisions of the ACA, and rejected it. First, the court noted the difficulty of distinguishing persuasion and coercion. The Eleventh Circuit also noted that after *Dole*, the Court had never devised a test to ascertain when financial pressure would lead to coercion, which had led many appeals courts to hold that the doctrine was not a viable defense to Spending Clause legislation.[46]

The Eleventh Circuit did, nonetheless, proceed to analyze whether the ACA Medicaid expansion had passed the point where "pressure turns into compulsion," and found that those provisions were not unduly coercive under

Dole. The court relied on a variety of factors. First, the Medicaid-participating states were warned from the beginning of the Medicaid program that Congress reserved the right to make changes to the program,[47] and since that time Congress had made numerous amendments to the program.[48] Second, most of the cost of the Medicaid expansion will be borne by the federal government until 2016, after which states will gradually become responsible for up to ten percent of the increase.[49]

Third, the court noted that the states would have nearly four years from the date the bill was signed into law to decide whether they will continue to participate in Medicaid, or, if they declined to do so, to develop a replacement program in their own states. Finally, the court noted that, under the Medicaid Act, HHS need not withhold all Medicaid funding to a state refusing to comply with the expansion, but it may withhold only a portion of such funding.[50]

The Supreme Court reversed the Eleventh Circuit, and held that the threat of withholding all Medicaid funding for failure to comply with the ACA Medicaid expansion was coercive, and so it violated the Tenth Amendment. The Supreme Court went on to hold, however, that to the extent that enforcement of the ACA Medicaid expansion through withdrawal of existing Medicaid funds was unconstitutional, that the remedy was to sever that enforcement mechanism. Based on both an explicit statutory severability clause[51] and on discernment of congressional intent,[52] the Court held that the Congress would have wanted the ACA Medicaid expansion to go forward. Thus the Court limited withholding of funds for failure to serve the expanded Medicaid population to withholding of those new funds, effectively making state participation in the Medicaid expansion voluntary.

As noted, the Supreme Court in *Dole* had identified two important factors in evaluating whether a congressional spending condition should be struck down under the Tenth Amendment – relatedness and coercion. The *NFIB* decision seemed to have most explicitly focused on the issue of coercion, but strains of relatedness permeate the opinion. This is seen most clearly in the concern expressed by the Court as to whether the states, upon entering the original Medicaid program, had been given sufficient notice of the possibility that such a significant expansion of the program might be imposed as a condition of participation.

The specific question accepted for consideration by the Supreme Court in *NFIB* was whether the ACA "violates basic principles of federalism" by "coerc[ing]" states into accepting "onerous conditions" in violation of *Dole*.[53] It should also be noted that the Court granted argument on this issue despite the fact that the Eleventh Circuit upheld the Medicaid expansion; that no other circuit has struck down these provisions;[54] and that no similar spending provisions have been previously invalidated under the coercion theory.[55]

Justice Roberts did not suggest that the decision in *NFIB* was inconsistent with prior Supreme Court cases, although it can be argued that the cursory analysis of relatedness and coercion in *Dole*[56] were elaborated significantly by his opinion, and may have been in some ways modified. Further, as will be discussed later, it would appear that coercion and relatedness were treated as separate factors by the Court in *Dole*.[57] In *NFIB*, however, the concepts appear to have become closely intertwined, so that in some contexts, relatedness and coercion must be considered together, not separately.

This latter approach is not inconsistent with unconstitutional conditions cases in non-state contexts. Where conditions associated with a governmental benefit have been challenged by a private person or entity, the "fit" of the benefit condition to the stated governmental purpose has been considered to increase concerns regarding coercive governmental behavior. For instance, in *Nollan v. California Coastal Commission,*[58] the owners of beachfront property in California sought a permit to demolish a bungalow and replace it with a three-bedroom house. The permit was granted subject to the condition that the owners record an easement allowing the public to cross their property in order to reach the beach. The permit condition was challenged as a taking of property without the just compensation required by the Constitution.[59] The California government argued that the new construction would increase blockage of the view of the ocean, creating a psychological barrier to beach access, and that the easement was necessary to counter this effect.[60] The Court, however, evaluated whether the condition in question, providing "physical access," served the purpose put forward as the justification for the prohibition, since the remedy for losing visual "access" to the beach was to provide the more significant physical "access" to the beach. Thus, the Court found that, at least in the takings context, there must be a close "fit" between the purpose of the regulation and the burden imposed, and that the conditioning of the permit in this manner was unconstitutional.[61]

Relatedness

Justice Roberts' decision in *NFIB* appears to contemplate that when a court evaluates a grant condition, it must determine the relationship between that grant condition and the underlying grant program. It had been suggested previously that the more closely federal grant conditions on states are tied to the purpose of the grant, the less likely courts will be to find coercion.[62] While the Justice Roberts' opinion in *NFIB* did not explicitly establish such a relationship between relatedness and coercion, it did indicate that certain categories of grant conditions are more vulnerable to a constitutional challenge under the doctrine of coercion than others.

In evaluating this relationship, Justice Roberts discusses several types of grant conditions: 1) conditions directly related to the expenditure of federal funds (hereinafter "directly related conditions"); 2) conditions related to the policy goals underlying grants (hereinafter "indirectly related conditions)"; 3) conditions related to the goals of a "new and independent" grant program ("independent grant conditions"); and 4) grant conditions not-related to the policy goals of the underlying grant ("unrelated grand conditions"). It should be noted, however, that these categories are not presented by Justice Roberts systematically, but rather are identified explicitly or implicitly at various places in the opinion. Consequently, it is not clear if the above categories should be considered as an exclusive listing of all possible types of grant conditions; whether one or more of these are variants of the same category; or whether these categories may to some extent overlap. However, for purposes of this report, it would appear that once it is determined what type of grant condition is before the court, this will inform whether the grant condition is likely to be coercive or not.

For instance, Justice Roberts indicated that if a grant condition was directly related to the expenditure of federal funds, then it would appear that the condition will usually be constitutional under the Spending Clause. Second, if the grant condition is generally related to the policy goals of the underlying grant, then in most foreseeable cases, withdrawal of all the program funds would be constitutional under the Spending Clause and the Tenth Amendment. However, if the grant condition is for a new and independent program; the government threatens the funding of an existing program; and the withholding of federal funding represents a significant portion of a state's budget, then the condition would be coercive under the Tenth Amendment. Finally, if a grant condition is unrelated to the general policy goals of the underlying grant, then it is most likely unconstitutional under the Spending Clause.

Directly Related Conditions: Use of Federal Funds

It has long been suggested in unconstitutional conditions cases that there is a distinction to be made between grant conditions that limit how federal funds are used, and conditions that limit or direct how a recipient will act in activities that are separate from such expenditures. In effect, concerns about coercion are substantially diminished when there is a direct relationship between the activity being directly subsidized by the government and the conditions imposed. This line of reasoning appears to hold true regardless of whether the grant recipient is a state or a private individual or entity, and it would appear to include situations where federal dollars provide just a part of the funding for a program or activity.

For instance, in the case of *Rust v. Sullivan*,[63] a First Amendment free speech challenge was brought against regulations that prohibited health care providers who received federal funds under Title X (which provided funds for family-planning services) to engage in abortion advocacy and counseling in any program receiving these funds.[64] If persons or entities associated with Title X projects sought to engage in these activities, they were required to do so in "physically and financially separate" locations.[65] Based on this distinction, the Court rejected the challenge to these regulations, holding that the government was not denying a subsidy or benefit because of the exercise of a constitutional right, but was only requiring that the federal funds be used for the purposes required by the statute: "to support preventive family planning services, population research, infertility services, and other related medical, informational, and educational activities."[66] Unlike other less related statutes, the Court here seemed to find that the direct relationship between the federal benefit and the activity in question justified the First Amendment limitations.

As noted, this same distinction has been true for Tenth Amendment challenges to federal grants to states. When a state is voluntarily receiving and spending federal funds, it is generally required to comply with federal conditions on how those funds are to be spent. For instance, in *Oklahoma v. Civil Service Comm'n*,[67] the Court considered the validity of the Hatch Act as applied to the political activities of state officials whose employment was financed in whole or in part with federal funds. The state contended that the withholding of federal funds unless a state official was removed invaded its sovereignty in violation of the Tenth Amendment. Though finding that the United States did not have the power to regulate the local political activities of such state officials, the Court held that the federal government "does have power to fix the terms upon which its money allotments to states shall be disbursed."[68]

This distinction between conditions on spending federal funds and other grant conditions was confirmed by Justice Roberts in *NFIB*. Justice Roberts' opinion stated that Congress's authority to condition the receipt of funds on the states' complying with restrictions on the use of those funds was the "means by which Congress ensures that the funds are spent according to its view of the 'general Welfare.'"[69] Although not explicitly finding that such restrictions could never be unconstitutional, there appears to be no suggestion in *NFIB* or any previous case that a state could be relieved from compliance with federal conditions on how to spend federal grant funds based on the size of the federal program or the amount of funds that would be withheld from that program for a violation.

Although a survey of existing state grant programs is beyond the scope of this report, it would appear that many federal grant conditions are conditions either directing or limiting certain behaviors in programs or activities that are spending federal funds.[70] Under the above analysis, it would appear that these restrictions would not be amenable to constitutional challenge under the Tenth Amendment. With regard to adding new federal conditions to existing state programs using federal funds, relevant case law does not appear to make a distinction between directly related grant conditions imposed at the time of a grant program's inception and conditions imposed later.[71] Thus, adding grant conditions to existing programs or activities receiving federal funds appears to be unremarkable, and arguably would not be subject to significant Tenth Amendment challenge.

Indirectly Related Conditions: Meeting Similar Policy Goals

Under a *Dole* analysis, a court will first analyze whether a grant condition is sufficiently related to an underlying grant. This inquiry, however, appears to be highly deferential to Congress, so that if any reasonable relationship between the policy goals of a program and the policy goals of the grant condition can be discerned, then the grant condition will be upheld. As noted, the relationship in *Dole* between raising the drinking age to twenty-one and the withholding of transportation funds was that both were associated with the issue of transportation safety. One can suggest that the Court's resort to such a high level of generality in finding that a condition was related would indicate that the relatedness standard in *Dole* would in most cases be easy to meet.

Thus, in the *NFIB* case, one would expect the Court to have little problem finding that grant conditions directly related to Medicaid's purpose of providing medical treatment to disadvantaged populations would meet the standard set forth in *Dole*. At a minimum, the new benefits provided under the Medicaid expansion would appear more closely tied to the purposes of the Medicaid program than the 21-year-old drinking age was to the purpose of the federal highway transportation funds under *Dole*. Justice Ginsburg, in dissent, suggests that the relatedness of Medicaid and the Medicaid expansion is undeniable.[72]

Justice Roberts' opinion, however, did not directly address whether the policy goals of the Medicaid expansion or any previous Medicaid amendments were related to the policy goals of the existing Medicaid program. Rather, as discussed below, Justice Roberts' opinion explored the narrower question as to whether the Medicaid expansion was a "new and independent" program. While this analysis might be seen as a variant of the *Dole* relatedness standard, Justice Roberts did not make this point explicitly. However, the opinion did suggest that all prior grant conditions which had been added to Medicaid over the years since its inception were constitutional. This would imply that, under *Dole*, those previous grant conditions were generally related to the policy goals of the program to which they were attached.

As discussed by Justice Ginsburg in her dissent, since 1965, Congress has amended the Medicaid program on more than 50 occasions.[73] The most dramatic expansion occurred between 1988 and 1990, when Congress required participating states to include among their beneficiaries pregnant women with family incomes up to 133 percent of the federal poverty level; children up to age six at the same income levels; and children ages six to eighteen with family incomes up to 100 percent of the poverty level.[74] According to Justice Ginsburg, these amendments added millions of people to the Medicaid-eligible population.[75]

Justice Roberts, however, makes clear in his opinion that the 1988-1990 Medicaid expansion was not of such a degree as to raise concerns about coercion under *Dole*. In *NFIB*, Justice Roberts argues that this previous modification should not be considered a major change in the Medicaid program, because Medicaid had always provided health care for "families with dependent children." Justice Roberts also suggested that none of the other 50 amendments would fall into the same category as the ACA expansion.[76]

Although not an explicit holding of the Court, Justice Roberts' opinion would suggest that most changes to federal spending programs will not raise significant constitutional concerns. Many of the amendments to Medicaid imposed grant conditions that, if not met, would result in the loss of all Medicaid funding.[77] And, as will be discussed later, Medicaid funding represents one of the largest federal programs providing money to the states. The suggestion of the Roberts' opinion is that even as significant a loss of federal funds as would occur with the withdrawal of federal Medicaid funding would pass constitutional muster, as long as the grant condition fell into the category of indirectly related conditions.

Independent Conditions: Requirement to Implement New Program

In *NFIB*, seven Justices held that the requirement that states either comply with the requirements of the Medicaid expansion under the ACA or lose all Medicaid funds violated the Tenth Amendment. However, these seven Justices either wrote or joined one of two separate opinions on this issue, and did not join in either the reasoning or judgment of the other opinion. The opinion of Chief Justice Roberts, which was joined by Justices Breyer and Kagan, appears to be significantly narrower than the dissenting opinion authored Justices Scalia, Kennedy, Thomas and Alito.[78] Thus, it would appear that for purposes of the Tenth Amendment challenge to the ACA, that the opinion by Chief Justice Roberts is the controlling opinion.[79]

The core of Justice Roberts' opinion is that the ACA Medicaid expansion creates a "new and independent" program, and that failure to comply with this new program will result in the withdrawal of funds for the existing Medicaid program. There were several aspects of the Medicaid expansion under the ACA that were deemed important in reaching this conclusion. It is unclear, however, whether all these factors needed to be present, or whether a challenge to a Spending Clause condition could be successful even if there had been less differentiation between Medicaid and this expansion. It does appear that the factors that were important in this case are unlikely to occur in other legislative contexts. Thus, if these factors mark the outer limits of Congress's power, then the case may have minimal impact on existing or future funding grant conditions.

Justice Roberts' opinion notes that Congress's power under the Spending Clause has been repeatedly characterized as "much in the nature of a contract,"[80] meaning that the states voluntarily and knowingly enter into an agreement with the federal government in order to receive federal funds. Previously, the significance of this theory has gone to the issue of statutory interpretation, so that conditions imposed on the states generally need to be explicit, and that the Supreme Court will presume against the creation of "implicit" conditions under the Spending Clause.

In Justice Roberts' opinion, however, the "contract" analogy serves a different purpose. In arguing that the Medicaid expansion should be viewed as a modification of an existing program, the United States noted that the original Medicaid program, found in the Social Security Act, contained a clause expressly reserving "[t]he right to alter, amend, or repeal any provision" of that statute.[81] However, Justice Roberts' opinion found that under the "contract" theory, the changes imposed by the Medicaid expansion were not of the type that were contemplated by the statute. Specifically, Justice Roberts' opinion indicated that the Medicaid expansion "accomplishes a shift in kind, not merely degree."[82]

The opinion noted that the original program had required states to cover medical services for four categories of persons in financial need: the disabled, the blind, the elderly, and needy families with dependent children.[83] Although previous amendments to Medicaid had altered the scope of these categories, the Medicaid expansion arguably changed the nature of the program by requiring recipient states to meet the health care needs of the entire nonelderly population with income below 133 percent of the poverty level. According to the opinion, this change meant the program was no longer to provide care for the neediest, but rather was an element of a comprehensive national plan to provide universal health care.[84]

Justice Roberts also wrote that the way this new Medicaid population is treated is different from how the existing Medicaid program works. For instance, under the ACA, Congress created a separate funding provision to cover the costs of providing services to any person made newly eligible by the expansion. While Congress pays 50 – 83 percent of the costs of covering individuals currently enrolled in Medicaid, once the expansion is fully implemented, Congress will pay 90 percent of the costs for newly eligible persons. Congress also mandated, however, that newly eligible persons would receive a level of coverage that is less comprehensive than the traditional Medicaid benefit package.[85]

In essence, Justice Roberts seems to have found that the states received insufficient notice upon their commitment to Medicaid that they might be required, as a condition of continuing in that program, to include significant new populations in their Medicaid coverage.[86] Despite the language in the Social Security Act regarding possible future alterations, the opinion found that this language did not confer on Congress the authority to transform the program so dramatically.

Unrelated Conditions: Does Not Address Similar Policy Goals

Justice Roberts indicated that, under *Dole*, if a Court finds that a policy goal is unrelated to the underlying grant condition, then that grant condition will not survive constitutional scrutiny under the Spending Clause.[87] After *Dole*, however, those lower courts that have considered relatedness challenges to grant conditions[88] do not appear to have engaged in particularly close scrutiny of this requirement.[89] In fact, some courts have even expressed a reluctance to engage in such an inquiry at all, suggesting that the difficulty of the analysis and the ability of states to seek relief through the political process precluded meaningful review.[90]

The question arises as to whether *NFIB* significantly affects this prong of the *Dole* analysis, so that lower courts would be likely to increase scrutiny of the relatedness requirement. It might be argued that the Roberts' opinion, with its emphasis on "new and independent" programs, is implicitly addressing the "relatedness" inquiry of *Dole*. Justice Roberts' opinion, however, does not explicitly discuss whether the "new and independent" grant condition analysis was intended to be considered separately from a relatedness inquiry; whether this analysis is a variant of the relatedness inquiry; or whether it was intended to supplant it.

An argument can be made, however, that there is a significant difference between the *Dole* "relatedness" inquiry and the *NFIB* "new and independent" program inquiry. First, as noted, the "relatedness inquiry" in *Dole* was identified as a limitation on the Spending Clause, while the *NFIB* discussion of "new and independent programs" emphasized the concerns of the Tenth Amendment. Second, under *Dole,* the "relatedness" and "coercion" inquiries appear to be disjunctive, in that failure to comply with either of these factors would mean that the statute was unconstitutional. Under *NFIB,* however (as is discussed below), the "new and independent program" inquiry and the "coercion" inquiry are conjunctive, so that a grant condition must apparently fail both tests to be found unconstitutional. If the *NFIB* analysis were either a supplement to or a replacement for the *Dole* "relatedness" doctrine, that doctrine would be significantly narrowed.

It would seem premature, without further clarification by the Court, for a lower court to apply such a limiting rule of construction to *Dole* (requiring challenges to successfully challenge both "relatedness" and "coercion"). Thus, arguably, the *Dole* "relatedness" test was not directly at issue in *NFIB*, and it is still the case that an unrelated grant condition will be found unconstitutional under the Spending Clause without the further requirement that such a condition be coercive. However, as noted previously, no federal statute has every been found by any court to fail under this requirement.

Coercion

When Coercion Analysis is Important

As suggested above, there are four types of grant conditions recognized by the Court: "Directly Related Conditions," "Indirectly Related Conditions,"

"Independent Program Conditions," and "Unrelated Program Conditions." And, as discussed above, a coercion analysis may not be particularly important for three of them. "Directly Related Conditions" are likely to be upheld and "Unrelated Conditions" conditions are likely to fail regardless of the level of funds withheld. Since, under *Dole* and *NFIB*, a coercion analysis still exists for "Indirectly Related" conditions, the implicit approval of Justice Roberts' opinion to the withholding of all Medicaid funding for the many amendments to Medicaid prior to the ACA makes it unlikely that past or future "Indirectly Related Conditions" will be constitutionally infirm. Thus, it would appear that only when a court ascertains that a grant condition associated with an "Independent Program Condition" is used to withhold existing funds that coercion analysis is likely to be relevant.

How Much Federal Funding Can be Withheld

Prior to *NFIB*, the Supreme Court had noted the inherent difficulty in determining when a state was being "coerced." In *Steward Machine Co. v. Davis*,[91] a corporation challenged a provision of the then newly enacted Social Security Act, arguing that the federal government had improperly coerced states into participation in the Social Security program. The Supreme Court rejected this argument, stating that:

> [T]o hold that motive or temptation is equivalent to coercion is to plunge the law in endless difficulties. The outcome of such a doctrine is the acceptance of a philosophical determinism by which choice becomes impossible. Till now the law has been guided by a robust common sense which assumes the freedom of the will as a working hypothesis in the solution of its problems.... Nothing in the case suggests the exertion of a power akin to undue influence, if we assume that such a concept can ever be applied with fitness to the relations between state and nation. Even on that assumption the location of the point at which pressure turns into compulsion, and ceases to be inducement, would be a question of degree, at times, perhaps, of fact.[92]

Thus, in *Steward*, the Court declined to establish a bright line test, instead just finding that the law in question did not fall outside of an acceptable level of persuasion.[93]

In *NFIB*, Justice Roberts took a similar approach. Rather than establishing a standard by which future coercion cases are to be judged against, the opinion merely concluded that the economic burden imposed by the withdrawal of all federal Medicaid funds would cross the line into coercion. Although the level of Medicaid expenditures in relationship to particular state budgets may vary, Justice Roberts characterized such levels as "the threatened loss of over 10 percent of a State's overall budget." Justice Roberts contrasted this amount with the amount of federal transportation funds threatened to be withheld in *Dole*, which Justice Roberts characterized as "less than half of one percent" of South Dakota's budget. Justice Roberts noted that the level of withdrawal of funds in *Dole* left that state with the "prerogative" to reject Congress's desired policy, "not merely in theory but in fact."[94] The loss of ten percent of a state's budget, on the other hand, represents a "gun to the head"[95] and a form of "economic dragooning"[96] which leaves the state no real option but to agree to the Medicaid expansion. How courts are to consider grant withdrawals between ten percent and one half of one percent, however, is not addressed by the Roberts' opinion, and Justice Roberts declined to speculate where such a line would be drawn.[97]

Justice Roberts' failure to "draw a line" in *NFIB* would seem, on its face, to make future predictions regarding grants conditions problematic. Medicaid is one of the largest federal programs currently in existence, and consequently, withdrawal of all Medicaid funds for failure to meet the Medicaid expansion requirements under the ACA would be disruptive to state finances. It is not clear, however, how the court might compare the levels of withdrawal threatened under the ACA from a variety of other large federal programs. It should be noted that, prior to the Court's decision in *NFIB*, various federal courts of appeals had considered and rejected coercion claims with respect to grants for state prisons,[98] education,[99] welfare,[100] and transportation.[101]

Whether Cost of Complying with Conditions is Relevant

One additional question that may be asked is whether a court should analyze the burden of compliance imposed by a federal grant condition as part of a coercion analysis. This question was considered an important part of the challenge to the Medicaid expansion – whether the grant condition in question was financially "onerous." In general, analysis under *Dole* has focused on the amount of federal funds withheld. In *NFIB*, however, the states argued that the Court should also consider the additional amounts of money that the states would have to expend to comply with the ACA Medicaid requirements.

The Court in *Dole* did not indicate that a coercion analysis varied based on the existence of a high burden of compliance (financially "onerous" or otherwise) imposed on the states by a grant condition. Instead, the Court appeared to focus its analysis on whether the grant condition in question threatened South Dakota's sovereignty and its ability to make its own policy decisions.[102] Arguably, the Court's decision in *Dole* would suggest that any grant condition that was "coercive" and intruded on a state's sovereignty would be unconstitutional, regardless of whether the financial or other burden of compliance was substantial or insignificant.[103] In either instance, the withdrawal of too much federal funding could have a coercive effect.[104]

In *NFIB,* Justice Roberts appears to have confirmed the implication of *Dole* – that the burdens of compliance are not a factor to be considered in a Tenth Amendment challenge to a federal spending condition. In a footnote, Justice Roberts summarily adopts this reasoning, noting that:

> [t]the size of the new financial burden imposed on a State is irrelevant in analyzing whether the State has been coerced into accepting that burden. "Your money or your life" is a coercive proposition, whether you have a single dollar in your pocket or $500.[105]

Thus, arguably, relatively minor grant conditions which involve the expenditure of some state funds (either directly or as administrative costs),[106] would still be subject to a coercion analysis.

CONCLUSION

The successful federalism challenge to Medicaid expansion under the ACA in the case of *NFIB* required the Supreme Court to address whether states are being "coerced" into compliance with the expanded state requirements by the threat of withholding existing Medicaid reimbursements. This "coercion" test, articulated in *South Dakota v. Dole* in 1987*,* had never been applied by the Supreme Court or the lower federal courts to strike down a federal statute, and had been so little developed by the Court that most federal courts of appeals had simply rejected similar challenges with little analysis. It is unclear, however, whether *NFIB* has significantly changed the *Dole* analysis, or whether the combination of factors that led to the Court's decision to limit how the ACA Medicaid expansion would be enforced is likely to be repeated.

As noted, Justice Roberts' decision in *NFIB* seems to contemplate the existence of several types of grant conditions: 1) conditions directly related to the expenditure of federal funds; 2) conditions related to the policy goals underlying grant; 3) conditions related to the goals of a "new and independent" grant program; and 4) grant conditions not related to the policy goals of the underlying grant.

Categories 1, 2 and 4 (direct, indirect, and unrelated conditions) are derived principally from prior case law, while category 3 (new and independent programs) appears to be the principal focus of *NFIB*. Prior case law holds (and *NFIB* confirms) that if a grant condition is directly related to the expenditure of federal funds in a state program or activity, then the condition is constitutional under the Spending Clause. Second, if the grant condition is generally related to the policy goals of the underlying grant, then, under *Dole* and *NFIB,* withdrawal of all program funds would, in most foreseeable cases, be constitutional under the Spending Clause and the Tenth Amendment. However, if the grant condition is attached to a new and independent program; the government threatens the funding of an existing program; and the withholding of federal funding represents a significant portion of a state's budget, then that condition may be unconstitutionally coercive under the Tenth Amendment. Finally, if a grant condition is unrelated to the general policy goals of the underlying grant, then it is most likely unconstitutional under the Spending Clause.

Thus, to the extent that a coercion remains relevant after *NFIB*, it would appear to apply principally where there is an existing program, and states are mandated to adopt a new and independent program at the risk of the state losing the existing funds. In this case, a court will need to consider whether the loss of funds for failure to adopt this new and independent program is coercive. Justice Roberts did not identify a standard to determine what level of funding withholding would be coercive, although he did conclude that withdrawal of federal program funds which represents ten percent of an average state's budget constituted a "gun to the head" and was a form of "economic dragooning." How courts are to consider grant withdrawals below ten percent, however, is not addressed by the Roberts opinion, and Justice Roberts declined to speculate where such a line would be drawn.

Finally, to the extent that such a new and independent program is found to be coercively mandated, then a court would need to fashion a remedy. In Justice Roberts' opinion, the Tenth Amendment remedy was not to strike down the "new and independent programs" (the ACA Medicaid expansion), but to disallow the threat of withholding existing funds (Medicaid). Based on both an explicit statutory severability clause and on discernment of congressional intent, the Court held that Congress would have wanted to preserve the authority to withhold funds from the expanded Medicaid population for failure to comply with its conditions. This ultimately had the effect of allowing the ACA Medicaid expansion to go forward, but effectively made state participation voluntary.

End Notes

[1] P.L. 111-148.

[2] P.L. 111-152.

[3] For background on the ACA, see CRS Report R41664, ACA: A Brief Overview of the Law, Implementation, and Legal Challenges, coordinated by C. Stephen Redhead.

[4] For a detailed analysis of these legal issues, see CRS Report R40725, Requiring Individuals to Obtain Health Insurance: A Constitutional Analysis, by Jennifer Staman et al..

[5] No. 11-393, slip op. (June 28, 2012). The states joining the suit include Alabama, Alaska, Arizona, Colorado, Florida, Georgia, Idaho, Indiana, Iowa, Kansas, Louisiana, Maine, Michigan, Mississippi, Nebraska, Nevada, North Dakota, Ohio, Pennsylvania, South Carolina, South Dakota, Texas, Utah, Washington, Wisconsin, and Wyoming. See Florida v. Dept. of Health and Human Services, 648 F.3d 1235, 1240 n.2 (11th Cir. 2011).

[6] For background on Medicaid, see CRS Report RL33202, Medicaid: A Primer, by Elicia J. Herz.

[7] For a detailed discussion of these provisions, see CRS Report R41210, Medicaid and the State Children's Health Insurance Program (CHIP) Provisions in ACA: Summary and Timeline, by Evelyne P. Baumrucker et al..

[8] 42 U.S.C. §1396a.

[9] 42 U.S.C. §1396a(a)(10)(A)(i)(VIII).

[10] States currently must provide Medicaid to children under age 6 with family income up to 133 percent of the FPL and children ages 6 through 18 with family income up to 100 percent of the FPL. 42 U.S.C. §§1396a(a)(10)(A)(i)(IV), (VI), (VII), 1396a(l)(1)(B)-(D), 1396a(l)(2)(A)-(C).

[11] Letter from Douglas Elmendorf, Director, Cong. Budget Office, to the Hon. Nancy Pelosi, Speaker, U.S. House of Reps. ("CBO Estimate") 9 (Mar. 20, 2010) cited in Petition for Writ of Certiorari, brief at 9-10, Florida v. HHS, No. 11-400 (Sept. 27, 2011)("Petitioner's Writ").

[12] CBO Estimate, Table 4.

[13] Kaiser Comm'n on Medicaid & the Uninsured, Medicaid Coverage & Spending in Health Reform: National and State-by-State Results for Adults at or Below 133% FPL at 23 (May 2010) (estimating that increased costs could be as high as $532 billion for federal government and $43.2 billion for states) cited in Petitioner's Writ at 9-10.

[14] The states note that, in the past, when Congress sought to expand Medicaid coverage, it offered additional funding to states that agreed to additional obligations, without threatening existing funding of states that did not. Petitioner's Writ. at 22. See, e.g., American Recovery and Reinvestment Act of 2009, P.L. 111-5, §5001(f); Omnibus Budget Reconciliation Act of 1986, P.L. 99-509, §9401(b).

[15] U.S. Const., Art. I, §8, cl. 1 ("The Congress shall have Power to lay and collect Taxes, Duties, Imposts and Excises, to pay the Debts and provide for the common Defence and general Welfare of the United States....").

[16] See United States v. Lopez, 514 U.S. 549 (1995) (striking down the Gun-Free School Zone Act of 1990).

[17] See New York v. United States, 505 U.S. 144 (1992) (striking down provisions of the Low-Level Radioactive Waste Policy Amendments Act of 1985); Printz v. United States, 521 U.S. 898 (1997) (striking down provisions of the Brady Handgun Control Act).

[18] See Seminole Tribe of Florida v. Florida, 517 U.S. 44 (1996) (Indian tribe may not sue state in federal court under the Indian Gaming Regulatory Act).

[19] See, e.g., 20 U.S.C. §1681 (1994) (prohibiting sex discrimination); 29 U.S.C. §794 (1994 & Supp. V 1999) (prohibiting discrimination on the basis of disability); 42 U.S.C. §§2000d to 2000d-4a (1994) (prohibiting race discrimination).

[20] See, e.g., New York, 505 U.S. at 188 (pointing out that the Spending Clause provides an alternative to the congressional "commandeering" of state officials that violated the Tenth Amendment); Lynn A. Baker, Conditional Federal Spending After Lopez, 95 Colum. L. Rev. 1911, 1914 (1995) ("Thus, with Dole, the Court offered Congress a seemingly easy end run around any restrictions the Constitution might impose on its ability to regulate the states.").

[21] Thus, in National League of Cities v. Usery, 426 U.S. 833 (1976), the Court struck down federal wage and price controls on state employees as involving the regulation of core state functions. In National League of Cities, the Court conceded that the legislation under attack, which regulated the wages and hours of certain state and local government employees, was within the scope of the Commerce Clause, but it cautioned that there are attributes of sovereignty attaching to every state government which may not be impaired by Congress, not because Congress may lack an affirmative grant of legislative authority to reach the matter, but because the Constitution prohibits it from exercising the authority in that manner.

[22] Garcia v. San Antonio Metropolitan Transit Authority, 469 U.S. 528 (1985). Justice Blackmun's opinion for the Court in Garcia concluded that the National League of Cities test for "integral operations" in areas of traditional governmental functions had proven impractical, and that the Court in 1976 had "tried to repair what did not need repair." 469 U.S. at 557. In sum, the Court in Garcia seems to have said that most disputes over the effects on state sovereignty of federal commerce power legislation are to be considered political questions. See also South Carolina v. Baker, 485 U.S. 505 (1988).

[23] 505 U.S. 144 (1992).

[24] Low-Level Radioactive Waste Policy Amendments Act of 1985, P.L. 99-240.

[25] 505 U.S. at 175-76.

[26] 521 U.S. 898 (1997).

[27] Brady Handgun Violence Prevention Act, P.L. 103-159, §102.

[28] 521 U.S. at 935.

[29] See Gilmore v. Utah, 429 U.S. 1012, 1014-16 (1976) (finding that the prisoner knowingly and intelligently waived his rights).

[30] See Brady v. United States, 397 U.S. 742, 748 (1970). In modern criminal practice, the right to a jury trial is often bargained away by a defendant in order to be allowed to plead guilty to lesser charges.

[31] Erwin Chemerinsky, CONSTITUTIONAL LAW: PRINCIPLES AND POLICIES at 798 (1997) ("[P]erhaps the cases cannot be reconciled, and the decisions simply turn on the views of the Justices in particular cases. If the Court wishes to strike down a condition, it declares it to be an unconstitutional condition; if the Court wishes to uphold a condition, it declares that the government is making a permissible choice to subsidize some activities and not others.").

[32] Angel D. Mitchell, Conditional Federal Funding to the States: The New Federalism Demands a Close Examination for Unconstitutional Conditions, 48 Kan. L. Rev. 161, 176 (1999).

[33] "The Supreme Court not only requires that the exchange be in some sense 'like kind,' but that the exchange be fair so that the foregone right is not in some sense disproportionate." Daniel A. Farber, Another View of the Quagmire: Unconstitutional Conditions and Contract Theory, 33 Florida State University L. Rev.913 (2003).

[34] Richard Epstein, Unconstitutional Conditions, State Power and the Limits of Consent, 102 Harv. L. Rev. 5, 21-22 (1988).

[35] Pace v. Bogalusa City School Bd., 403 F.3d 272, 286 (5th Cir. 2005). However, as is discussed later, the more related the condition is to the underlying federal benefit, the more reluctant the courts has been to find that the constitutional right is being "coerced."

[36] NFIB, slip op. at 47 (Ginsburg, J., dissenting).

[37] 483 U.S. 203 (1987).

[38] National Minimum Drinking Age Amendment of 1984, 23 U.S.C. §158.

[39] U.S. Const., Art I, §8, cl. 1 (Congress has the power to "lay and collect Taxes, Duties, Imposts, and Excises, to pay the Debts and provide for the common Defence and general Welfare of the United States").

[40] The Court easily dispensed with two preliminary questions. First, it held that the law was consistent with the requirements of Article I, §8, cl. 3 that spending be "in pursuit of 'the general welfare.'" Second, it held that a requirement that the condition be unambiguous so that states can make choices knowingly and be aware of the consequences was met. Dole, 483 U.S. at 207 (citing Helvering v. Davis, 301 U.S. 619, 640-41 (1937); United States v. Butler, 297 U.S. 1, 65 (1936)).

[41] 483 U.S. at 207.

[42] See 483 U.S. at 208.

[43] 483 U.S. at 208.

[44] 483 U.S. at 211.

[45] Florida v. HHS, 648 F.3d 1235 (11th Cir. 2011).

[46] See, e.g., Pace v. Bogalusa City School Bd., 403 F.3d 272, 278 (5th Cir. 2005) (en banc) ("It goes without saying that, because states have the independent power to lay and collect taxes, they retain the ability to avoid the imposition of unwanted federal regulation simply by rejecting federal funds."); A.W. v. Jersey City Pub. Schools, 341 F.3d 234, 243- 44 (3d Cir. 2003) (noting that the state's freedom to tax makes it difficult to find a federal law coercive, even when that law threatens to withhold all federal funding in a particular area); California v. United States, 104 F.3d 1086, 1092 (9th Cir. 1997) (noting in a Medicaid expansion case that "to the extent that there is any viability left in the coercion theory, it is not reflected in the facts of this record"); Nevada v. Skinner, 884 F.2d 445, 448 (9th Cir. 1989) ("The difficulty if not the impropriety of making judicial judgments regarding a state's financial capabilities renders the coercion theory highly suspect as a method for resolving disputes between federal and state governments.").

[47] See 42 U.S.C. §1304 ("The right to alter, amend, or repeal any provision of this chapter is hereby reserved to the Congress").

[48] For example, in 1972, Congress required participating states to extend Medicaid to recipients of Supplemental Security Income, thereby significantly expanding Medicaid enrollment. Social Security Act Amendments of 1972, Pub. L. No. 92-603, 86 Stat. 1329 (1972). In 1989, Congress again expanded enrollment by requiring states to extend Medicaid to pregnant women and children under age six who meet certain income limits. Omnibus Budget Reconciliation Act of 1989, P.L. 101-239, 103 Stat. 2106 (1989).

[49] 648 F.3d at 1267.

[50] 648 F.3d at 1286. See 42 U.S.C. §1396c.

[51] 42 U.S.C. §1396c ("If any provision of this chapter, or the application thereof to any person or circumstance, is held invalid, the remainder of the chapter, and the application of such provision to other persons or circumstances shall not be affected thereby.").

[52] NFIB, slip op at 57 ("We are confident that Congress would have wanted to preserve the rest of the Act. .... We have no way of knowing how many States will accept the terms of the expansion, but we do not believe Congress would have wanted the whole Act to fall, simply because some may choose not to participate.").

[53] Supreme Court Order List (November 14, 2011)(cert. granted to question: Does "Congress[s] exceed its enumerated powers and violate basic principles of federalism when it coerces States into accepting onerous conditions that it could not impose directly by threatening to withhold all federal funding under the single largest grant-in-aid program, or does the limitation on Congress's spending power that this Court recognized in South Dakota v. Dole, 483 U.S. 203 (1987), no longer apply?," Petitioner's Cert., at i).

[54] Generally, the criterion for the Supreme Court to take a case is that there is disagreement between federal circuit courts on an issue, or because a federal law has been struck down. Robert Stern, Eugene Gressman, Stephen Shapiro, SUPREME COURT PRACTICE at 194, 213 (6th Ed. 1986).

[55] See Nevada v. Skinner, 884 F.2d 445, 448-49 (9th Cir. 1989) ("The coercion theory has been much discussed but infrequently applied in federal case law, and never in favor of the challenging party.").

[56] The discussion of relatedness took two paragraphs, Dole, 483 U.S. at 207-09, while the discussion of coercion extended over slightly more than one page. Dole, 483 U.S. at 211 – 212.

[57] Dole, 483 U.S. at 207-09, 211-12.

[58] 483 U.S. 825 (1987).

[59] The Fifth Amendment (which has been incorporated against the states through the Fourteenth Amendment), provides that "nor shall private property be taken for public use, without just compensation."

[60] The Court noted that if California had merely taken the easement outright, this would have required payment of just compensation. On the other hand, the Court opined that the government's "power to forbid construction of the house in order to protect the public's view of the beach must surely include the power to condition construction upon some concession by the owner, even a concession of property rights, that serves the same end." 483 U.S. at 836.

[61] 483 U.S. at 838.

[62] See, e.g., Angel D. Mitchell, Conditional Federal Funding to the States: The New Federalism Demands a Close Examination for Unconstitutional Conditions, 48 Kan. L. Rev. 161 (1999); Virginia Department of Education v. Riley, 106 F.3d at 570 (en banc) (per curiam) (incorporating Judge Luttig's dissent from prior panel decision) (federal decision to withhold special education funds because of a state policy allowing suspension of special education students intrudes on disciplinary issues, an area of state, not federal, concern).

[63] 500 U.S. 173 (1991).

[64] 500 U.S. at 179-80.

[65] 500 U.S. at 180-81.

[66] H. R. Conf. Rep. No. 91-1667, at 8 (1970).

[67] 330 U. S. 127 (1947).

[68] 330 U.S. at 143.

[69] NFIB, slip op. at 50.

[70] See, e.g., note 19, supra (prohibiting discrimination in programs or activities receiving federal funds).

[71] See Bennett v. Kentucky Dept. of Ed., 470 U. S. 656, 659–660 (1985) (enforcing restriction added five years after adoption of educational program); NFIB, slip op. at 46 (Ginsburg, J., dissenting).

[72] NFIB, slip op. at 47-48 (Ginsburg, J., dissenting).

[73] NFIB, slip op. at 41-42 (Ginsburg, J., dissenting).

[74] See 42 U. S. C. §§1396a(a)(10)(A)(i), 1396a(l).

[75] NFIB, slip op. at 42 (Ginsburg, J., dissenting), citing DUBAY & KENNEY, Lessons from the Medicaid Expansions for Children and Pregnant Women 5 (Apr. 1997).

[76] NFIB, slip op. at 55.

[77] NFIB, slip op. at 53. Congress has sometimes conditione only new Medicaid funding, while at other time it has conditioned both old and new. See, e.g., Social Security Amendments of 1972, 86 Stat. 1381–1382, 1465 (extending Medicaid eligibility, but partly conditioning only the new funding); Omnibus Budget Reconciliation Act of 1990, §4601, 104 Stat. 1388–166 (extending eligibility, and conditioning old and new funds).

[78] While Justice Roberts, as discussed below, finds a constitutional violation based on the presence of both a "new and independent" program and a coercive loss of funds, the dissenting opinion would find the loss of federal funds a sufficient basis to strike down the ACA Medicaid expansion. NFIB, slip op. at 38-42 (Justices Scalia, Kennedy, Thomas and Alito dissenting).

[79] Marks v. United States, 430 U.S. 188, 193 (1977)("[w]hen a fragmented Court decides a case and no single rationale explaining the result enjoys the assent of five Justices, 'the holding of the Court may be viewed as that position taken by those Members who concurred in the judgments on the narrowest grounds'") (citation omitted).

[80] Barnes v. Gorman, 536 U. S. 181, 186 (2002); Pennhurst State School and Hospital v. Halderman, 451 U.S. 1, 17 (1981).

[81] 42 U.S.C. § 1304.

[82] NFIB, slip op. at 53.

[83] 42 U.S.C. §1396a(a)(10).

[84] NIFB, slip op. at 53-54.

[85] NFIB, slip op. at 54.

[86] Pennhurst, 451 U. S at 25 ("[t]hough Congress' power to legislate under the spending power is broad, it does not include surprising participating States with post acceptance or 'retroactive' conditions.").

[87] NFIB, slip op. at 50.

[88] See, e.g., Jim C. v. United States, 235 F.3d 1079, 1084 (8th Cir. 2000) (Bowman, J, dissenting) (arguing that waiver of sovereign immunity was not related to purpose of education grants).

[89] See, e.g., Pace v. Bogalusa City Sch. Bd., 403 F.3d 272, 287 (5th Cir. 2005) (en banc) (threatened loss of $800 million not coercive because state could have declined federal funds); A.W. v. Jersey City Pub. Sch., 341 F.3d 234, 255 (3d Cir. 2003) ("state's powers as a political sovereign, especially its authority to tax, appear more than capable of preventing undue coercion"); Jim C. v. United States, 235 F.3d 1079, 1082 (8th Cir. 2000) (en banc) (threatened loss of $250 million "politically painful," not coercive); California v. United States, 104 F.3d 1086, 1092 (9th Cir. 1997) (coercion "not reflected" by threatened loss of all Medicaid funding).

[90] See, e.g., Nevada v. Skinner, 884 F.2d 445, 448-49 (9th Cir. 1989) (coercion doctrine presents "questions of policy and politics that range beyond [the judiciary's] normal expertise" and should be discarded because states are "adequately protected by the national political process"); Kansas v. United States, 214 F.3d 1196, 1202 (10th Cir. 2000) (declaring doctrine "unclear" and "suspect").

[91] 301 U.S. 548 (1937).

[92] 301 U.S. at 589-90, 892 (quotation marks, citation omitted).

[93] 301 U.S. at 591.

[94] NFIB, slip op. at 51-52 (quoting Dole, 483 U. S. at 211–212.).

[95] NFIB, slip op. at 51.

[96] NFIB, slip op. at 52.

[97] NFIB, slip op. at 55.

[98] See, e.g., Van Wyhe v. Reisch, 581 F.3d 639, 652 (8th Cir. 2009), cert. denied, 130 S. Ct. 3323 (2010), and 131 S. Ct. 2149 (2011).

[99] See, e.g., Jim C. v. United States, 235 F.3d 1079, 1082 (8th Cir. 2000).

[100] See, e.g., Kansas v. United States, 214 F.3d 1196, 1198, 1201-1202 (10th Cir. 2000).

[101] See, e.g., Nevada v. Skinner, 884 F.2d 445, 448-449 (9th Cir. 1989).

[102] Dole, 483 U.S. at 211-212 (upholding the grant condition because "the enactment of such laws remains the prerogative of the States not merely in theory but in fact").

[103] This reasoning is bolstered by the Court's Tenth Amendment analysis, in which the Court rejected an argument that the level of the financial burden imposed by compliance with a federal directive was relevant to a finding of commandeering. In Printz, the federal government argued that the requirements imposed on state and local officials by the Brady Act were a "minimal [and] temporary burden." Printz, 521 U.S. at 932. The Court responded:

But where, as here, it is the whole object of the law to direct the functioning of the state executive, and hence to compromise the structural framework of dual sovereignty, such a "balancing" analysis is inappropriate. It is the very principle of separate state sovereignty that such a law offends, and no comparative assessment of the various interests can overcome that fundamental defect.

521 U.S. at 932-33.

[104] To the extent that the Court did decide to introduce an evaluation of the financial burden of compliance to its Dole analysis, one could argue that, rather than finding that a high or "onerous" level of burden is necessary to a finding of coercion, the Court might conclude that states' were more likely to be coerced when the burden of compliance was relatively insubstantial. See Virginia Department of Education v. Riley, 106 F.3d 559 (4th Cir. 1997) (en banc) (per curiam) (incorporating Judge Luttig's dissent from prior panel decision).

[105] NFIB, slip op. at 52 n 12.

[106] Id.

In: Medicaid Expansion …
Editor: Gail Norman
ISBN: 978-1-63463-442-7

Chapter 3

MISSED OPPORTUNITIES: THE CONSEQUENCES OF STATE DECISIONS NOT TO EXPAND MEDICAID*

The Council of Economic Advisers

SUMMARY AND INTRODUCTION

The Affordable Care Act has expanded high-quality, affordable health insurance coverage to millions of Americans. One important way in which the Affordable Care Act is expanding coverage is by providing generous financial support to States that opt to expand Medicaid eligibility to all non-elderly individuals in families with incomes below 133 percent of the Federal Poverty Level.

To date, 26 States and the District of Columbia have seized this opportunity, and since the beginning of the Affordable Care Act's first open enrollment period, 5.2 million people have gained Medicaid or Children's Health Insurance Program (CHIP) coverage in these States, a tally that will grow in the months and years ahead as Medicaid enrollment continues. In contrast, 24 States have not yet expanded Medicaid—including many of the States that would benefit most and sometimes because State legislatures have defied even their own governors—and denied health insurance coverage to

* This is an edited, reformatted and augmented version of a report issued by the Executive Office of the President, July 2014.

millions of their citizens. Researchers at the Urban Institute estimate that, if these States do not change course, 5.7 million people will be deprived of health insurance coverage in 2016. Meanwhile, these States will forgo billions in Federal dollars that could boost their economies.

This analysis uses the best evidence from the economics and health policy literatures to quantify several important consequences of States' decisions not to expand Medicaid. That evidence, which is based primarily on careful analysis of the effects of past policy decisions, is necessarily an imperfect guide to the future, and the actual effects of Medicaid expansion under the Affordable Care Act could be larger or smaller than the estimates presented below. However, this evidence is clear that the consequences of States' decisions are far-reaching, with implications for the health and well-being of their citizens, their economies, and the economy of the Nation as a whole.

DIRECT BENEFITS OF EXPANDED INSURANCE COVERAGE FOR THE NEWLY INSURED

One direct consequence of States' decisions not to expand Medicaid is that millions of their uninsured citizens will not experience the improved access to health care, greater financial security, and better health outcomes that come with insurance coverage.

Improved Access to Care

Having health insurance improves access to health care. This analysis estimates that if the States that have not yet expanded Medicaid did so:

- 1.4 million more people would have a usual source of clinic care.

Having health insurance increases the probability that individuals have a usual source of clinic care, like a primary care physician's office. If the 24 States that have not yet expanded Medicaid did so, an additional 1.4 million people would have a usual source of clinic care once expanded coverage was fully in effect. States that have already expanded Medicaid will achieve this outcome for 1.0 million people.

- 651,000 more people would receive all care they feel they need in a typical year.

Having health insurance increases the probability that individuals report receiving “all needed care” over the prior year. If the 24 States that have not yet expanded Medicaid did so, an additional 651,000 people would receive “all needed care” over a given year once expanded coverage was fully in effect. States that have already expanded Medicaid will achieve this outcome for 494,000 people.

- Hundreds of thousands more people would receive recommended preventive care each year.

Having health insurance increases the probability of receiving many types of recommended and potentially life-saving preventive care, including:

- Cholesterol-level screenings: If the 24 States that have not yet expanded Medicaid did so, then each year an additional 829,000 people would receive cholesterol-level screenings once expanded coverage was fully in effect. States that have already expanded Medicaid will achieve this outcome for 630,000 people.
- Mammograms: If the 24 States that have not yet expanded Medicaid did so, then each year an additional 214,000 women between the ages of 50 and 64 would receive mammograms once expanded coverage was fully in effect. States that have already expanded Medicaid will achieve this outcome for 161,000 women in this age group.
- Papanicolaou tests (“pap smears”): If the 24 States that have not yet expanded Medicaid did so, then each year an additional 345,000 women would receive pap smears once expanded coverage was fully in effect. States that have already expanded Medicaid will achieve this outcome for 261,000 women.

- Millions of people would be better able to obtain other needed medical care.

Having health insurance also increases receipt of other types of medical care. For example, if the 24 States that have not yet expanded Medicaid did so, they would enable an additional 15.4 million physician office visits each year once expanded coverage was fully in effect. States that have already expanded

Medicaid will enable an additional 11.7 million physician office visits each year.

Greater Financial Security

Having health insurance provides protection from financial hardship in the face of sickness. This analysis estimates that if the States that have not yet expanded Medicaid did so:

- 255,000 fewer people will face catastrophic out-of-pocket medical costs in a typical year.

High-quality health insurance coverage dramatically reduces the risk that individuals face catastrophic out-of-pocket medical costs (defined as costs in excess of 30 percent of income). If the 24 States that have not yet expanded Medicaid did so, 255,000 fewer people would face catastrophic medical costs each year once expanded coverage was fully in effect. States that have already expanded Medicaid will eliminate catastrophic medical costs for 194,000 people each year.

- 810,000 fewer people will have trouble paying other bills due to the burden of medical costs.

Having health insurance reduces individuals' risk of having to borrow money to pay bills or skip a payment entirely in order to pay medical bills. If the 24 states that have not yet expanded Medicaid did so, 810,000 fewer people would report this type of financial strain over the course of a year once expanded coverage was fully in effect. States that have already expanded Medicaid will achieve this outcome for 614,000 people each year.

Better Mental Health

Having insurance improves mental health. This analysis estimates that if the 24 States that have not yet expanded Medicaid did so, there would be 458,000 fewer people experiencing depression once expanded coverage was fully in effect. States that have already expanded Medicaid will reduce the number of people experiencing depression by 348,000.

Better Overall Health

Having insurance coverage improves overall health. This analysis estimates that if the 24 States that have not yet expanded Medicaid did so, 757,000 additional people would report being in excellent, very good, or good health once expanded coverage was fully in effect. States that have already expanded Medicaid will achieve this outcome for 575,000 people.

BENEFITS OF EXPANDING MEDICAID FOR STATE ECONOMIES

Healthier workers who are less financially stressed and in better mental health may be more likely to participate in the workforce or have higher productivity on the job, economic benefits that could be important over the long run. More immediately, States that fail to expand Medicaid are also passing up billions of Federal dollars that could boost their economies today. By increasing low-income individuals' ability to access care, relieving cash-strapped families of high out-of-pocket costs, and reducing uncompensated care, the expansion in insurance coverage enabled by those Federal dollars would boost demand for medical and non-medical goods and services. Over the next few years, while the recovery from the 2007-2009 recession remains incomplete and slack remains in the economy, this increase in demand would boost overall employment and economic activity.

This analysis estimates that expanding Medicaid would generate the following benefits for States' economies today:

Additional Federal Funds

By expanding Medicaid, States can pull billions in additional Federal funding into their economies every year, with no State contribution over the next three years and only a modest one thereafter for coverage for newly eligible people. If the 24 States that have not yet expanded Medicaid had done so as of January 1, those States and their citizens would have received an additional $88 billion in Federal support through calendar year 2016. States that have already expanded Medicaid will receive $84 billion over that period.

More Jobs

By pumping more Federal dollars into their economies, States' decisions to expand Medicaid create jobs. If the 24 States that have not yet expanded Medicaid had done so as of January 1, they would have boosted employment by 85,000 jobs in 2014, 184,000 jobs in 2015, and a total of 379,000 job-years through 2017. States that have already expanded Medicaid will boost employment by 79,000 jobs in 2014, 172,000 jobs in 2015, and a total of 356,000 job-years through 2017.

Greater Overall Economic Activity

By pumping more Federal dollars into their economies, States' decisions to expand Medicaid increase the overall level of economic activity. If the 24 States that have not yet expanded Medicaid had done so as of January 1, they would have created an additional $66 billion in total economic activity through 2017. States that have already expanded Medicaid will create $62 billion in total economic activity through 2017.

The remainder of this report provides more detail on States' option to expand Medicaid under the Affordable Care Act, discusses the effects of States' choices for their uninsured citizens and their economies, presents the methodology used to quantify those effects, and provides tables and figures with State-by-State detail.

I. Background on States' Option to Expand Medicaid under the Affordable Care Act

Medicaid is a program jointly funded by the Federal government and the States that provides health insurance to eligible low-income people. Each State operates its own Medicaid program and has considerable flexibility in determining eligibility criteria. The Affordable Care Act (ACA) gives States the option to expand their Medicaid programs to all non-elderly individuals in families with incomes below 133 percent of the Federal Poverty Level (FPL). Program rules provide for an additional five percent "income disregard," bringing the effective eligibility threshold to 138 percent of FPL: $16,105 for a single adult or $32,913 for a family of four in 2014. Because children at these income levels are generally already eligible for Medicaid or the Children's Health Insurance Program, this expansion primarily affects low-income adults. Prior to the Affordable Care Act's Medicaid expansion, the median eligibility level for working parents was only 61 percent of the FPL, and, in nearly all States, non-disabled adults without children were not eligible at all (Heberlein et al. 2013). As depicted in Figure 1, as of July 2, 2014, 26 States and the District of Columbia had taken advantage of this option to expand their Medicaid programs.

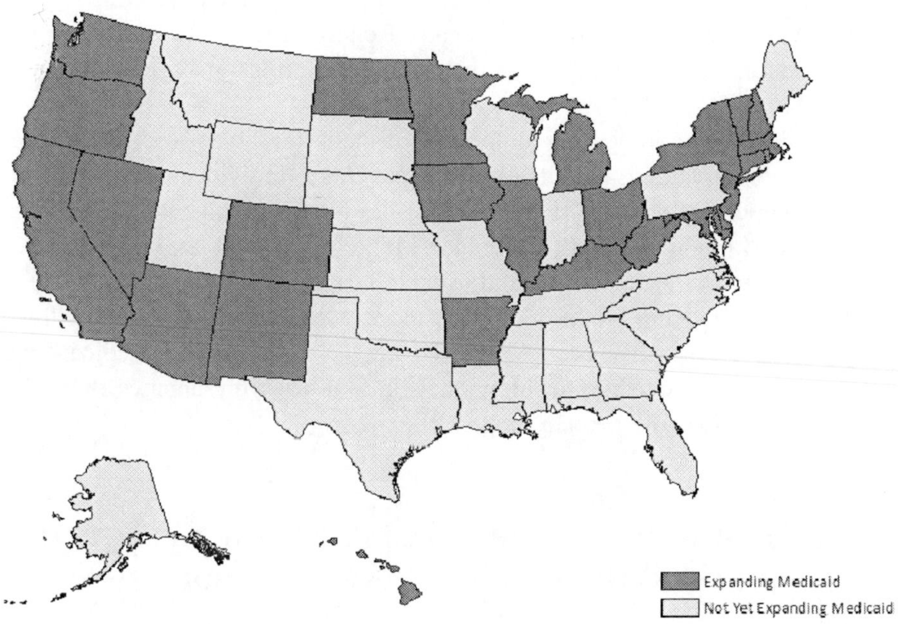

Figure 1. States Expanding and Not Yet Expanding Medicaid.

The Federal government will cover the vast majority of the costs of expanding Medicaid eligibility under the Affordable Care Act. Through 2016, the Federal government will pay 100 percent of the costs of covering newly eligible individuals, falling gradually to 90 percent in 2020 and subsequent years. This is a considerably larger Federal contribution than for eligibility categories in existence before the Affordable Care Act, for which program costs are shared between the Federal government and the States according to a formula that targets additional assistance to lower-income States, with the Federal share averaging around 57 percent and ranging from 50 percent to just under 74 percent in fiscal year 2014.[1]

States electing to expand their Medicaid programs are likely to realize large savings in other areas of their budgets that offset even the modest increase in State Medicaid spending after 2016. Researchers at the Urban Institute have estimated that, if all States expanded Medicaid, reductions in uncompensated care currently financed by State governments would more than offset any additional Medicaid costs, generating $10 billion in savings over ten years for all States, although the net impact will vary by State (Holahan, Buettgens, and Dorn 2013). That analysis also omits other potential State savings, including reduced costs to States of providing mental health services that would now be covered by Medicaid. Related research by some of these same authors has concluded that these other savings may be substantial (Buettgens et al. 2011).

Medicaid is an important component of the Affordable Care Act's overall approach to expanding health insurance coverage. Individuals with incomes under 100 percent of the FPL are not eligible for tax credits and cost-sharing assistance through the Health Insurance Marketplaces and, as a consequence, will generally not have access to affordable health insurance coverage if their State does not expand Medicaid. Furthermore, Medicaid typically offers lower out-of-pocket costs than Marketplace coverage, so expanding Medicaid will lower the cost of coverage for individuals in families with incomes above 100 percent and below 138 percent of the FPL.

II. Methodology for Estimating the Effects of States' Decisions to Expand Medicaid

To estimate the consequences of State decisions to expand Medicaid, this analysis proceeds in two steps. First, CEA obtained estimates of States' Medicaid expansion decisions on insurance coverage and the amount of Federal funding entering State economies; these estimates were either taken directly from or derived from publications by the Urban Institute and the Congressional Budget Office. Second, CEA used research on the effects of past policy decisions to translate those direct effects into impacts on the ultimate outcomes of interest: access to care, financial security, health and well-being, and the Nation's economic performance.

The available research literature unambiguously demonstrates that State decisions to expand Medicaid will have large effects in all of these areas, effects that are reflected in the estimates reported in this analysis. Nevertheless, it is important to keep in mind that, while all of the studies this report draws upon are rigorous, all research has limitations. Statistical analyses are subject to sampling errors, as well as other imperfections that can cause estimates to systematically overstate or understate the effects of the policy changes studied. In addition, the effects of past policy changes may not be a perfect guide to the effects of future policy changes. As a consequence, while the estimates presented in this analysis represent the best available estimates of the effects of expanding Medicaid, the actual effects could turn out to be larger or smaller than the estimates presented in this report.

The remainder of this section describes CEA's methodology in greater detail.

Effects on Insurance Coverage

The most direct consequence of State decisions to expand Medicaid is to increase insurance coverage in that State. Because the other benefits of expanding Medicaid flow from this basic effect, estimates of how expanding Medicaid affects insurance coverage are a crucial input into the rest of the analyses undertaken in this report. In this report, CEA relies upon published results from the Urban Institute's Health Insurance Policy Simulation Model (HIPSM), which provide State-by-State estimates of how each State's decision about whether to expand Medicaid would affect insurance coverage in that State (Holahan et al. 2012; Holahan, Buettgens, and Dorn 2013). The HIPSM national estimates of how the Affordable Care Act will affect insurance coverage are broadly similar to those produced by other analysts, including the Congressional Budget Office (CBO 2012a) and the RAND Corporation (Eibner et al. 2010).

Table 1. Increase in Number of People with Insurance Coverage if State Expands Medicaid

	People with Insurance Coverage in 2016
Not Yet Expanding Medicaid	**5,692,000**
Alabama	235,000
Alaska	26,000
Florida	848,000
Georgia	478,000
Idaho	55,000
Indiana	262,000
Kansas	100,000
Louisiana	265,000
Maine	28,000
Mississippi	165,000
Missouri	253,000
Montana	38,000
Nebraska	48,000
North Carolina	377,000
Oklahoma	123,000
Pennsylvania	305,000
South Carolina	198,000
South Dakota	26,000
Tennessee	234,000
Texas	1,208,000
Utah	74,000
Virginia	210,000
Wisconsin	120,000
Wyoming	16,000
Expanding Medicaid	**4,321,000**
Arizona	51,000
Arkansas	143,000
California	1,390,000
Colorado	154,000
Connecticut	84,000
Delaware	7,000
District of Columbia	19,000
Hawaii	39,000
Illinois	398,000
Iowa	20,000
Kentucky	177,000

Maryland	135,000
Massachusetts	2,000
Michigan	212,000
Minnesota	42,000
Nevada	105,000
New Hampshire	26,000
New Jersey	227,000
New Mexico	96,000
New York	167,000
North Dakota	21,000
Ohio	446,000
Oregon	186,000
Rhode Island	26,000
Vermont	4,000
Washington	64,000
West Virginia	80,000

Source: Urban Institute.

The HIPSM estimates show that, if all States expanded Medicaid, the number of people in the United States with insurance coverage would increase by 10 million by 2016, reflecting an increase of 4.3 million in the 26 States and the District of Columbia that have already expanded the program and an increase of 5.7 million in the 24 States that have yet do to so.[2] This report focuses on the HIPSM estimates for 2016 because these should provide a reasonable guide of the long-run effects of Medicaid expansion on insurance coverage, after the initial "ramp-up." Consistent with that, this analysis refers to these HIPSM estimates for 2016 as reflecting the effects of expanded Medicaid coverage "when fully in effect." The detailed State-by-State estimates are reported in Table 1.

Actual experience since the beginning of the Affordable Care Act's first open enrollment period has borne out model-based predictions that States' decisions about whether to expand Medicaid will have significant implications for insurance coverage. In the States (and the District of Columbia) that have expanded Medicaid, the number of people with health insurance coverage through Medicaid (or CHIP) has increased by 5.2 million (15.3 percent) from the third quarter of 2013 through April 2014 (CMS 2014).[3] By contrast, Medicaid enrollment in States that have not yet expanded Medicaid has risen by 0.8 million (3.3 percent) over that period. (The modest increase in Medicaid enrollment in states that have not yet expanded Medicaid is likely attributable to simplifications in Medicaid eligibility rules required of all

States and outreach, public awareness, and new enrollment options associated with the opening of the Marketplaces.)

Similarly, surveys have shown much larger increases in insurance coverage in States that have expanded Medicaid relative to states that have not. Comparing the third quarter of 2013 with early March 2014, the Urban Institute's Health Reform Monitoring Survey found a 4.0 percentage point increase in the percentage of non-elderly adults with insurance coverage in States that had expanded the program, compared to a 1.5 percentage point increase in States that had not done so (Long et al. 2014). Similarly, a survey by Gallup has found that States that expanded Medicaid and operated their own Marketplaces (alone or in partnership with the Federal government) experienced a 2.5 percentage point increase in the share of adults with insurance coverage from 2013 through the first quarter of 2014, compared with a 0.8 percentage point increase in States that have not taken these actions (Witters 2014).

Effects on Access to and Use of Medical Care

Perhaps the most obvious purpose of the Medicaid program is to ensure that enrollees have access to and receive needed medical care. To quantify the improvement in access to medical care that will results from States' decisions to expand Medicaid, this analysis relies upon estimates from the Oregon Health Insurance Experiment (Finkelstein et al. 2012; Baicker et al. 2013a; Baicker et al. 2013b; Taubman et al. 2014). The Oregon Health Insurance Experiment (OHIE) arose from the State of Oregon's decision in early 2008 to reopen enrollment under an earlier Medicaid expansion that had extended coverage to uninsured adults with incomes under 100 percent of the FPL. Because the State could not accommodate all interested applicants, it allocated the opportunity to enroll in Medicaid by lottery.

The State of Oregon's decision to allocate Medicaid coverage by lottery created a unique research opportunity. By comparing individuals who won the lottery to individuals who lost the lottery, it is possible to isolate the causal effect of having or not having Medicaid coverage, without the concern that the comparison is confounded by unobserved differences between those who do and do not have Medicaid coverage. Randomized research designs of this kind are considered the "gold standard" in social science research, and the OHIE is unique in using such a design to study the effects of having health insurance.

An additional important advantage of the OHIE for the current analysis is that the population that gained coverage in the Medicaid expansion studied in the OHIE—low-income, uninsured adults— is quite similar to the group that will gain health insurance coverage if States expand Medicaid under the Affordable Care Act. This increases the confidence that the results of the OHIE can be extrapolated to the Affordable Care Act's Medicaid expansion.

Of course, as noted at the outset, no study based on past policy changes in a specific environment applies perfectly to a future policy change in a different environment. Oregon's health care system differs from other States' health care systems in some ways, including the availability of medical providers (Huang and Finegold 2013), and other States' low-income populations do not look precisely like Oregon's. In addition, the OHIE can only speak to results over a follow-up period of approximately two years, but the effects of insurance coverage could differ over longer periods. Finally, the effects of larger-scale coverage expansions could differ from the effects of the smaller-scale expansion examined in the OHIE. Nevertheless, the OHIE clearly provides the best available estimates for quantifying many potential effects of States' decisions to expand Medicaid under the Affordable Care Act.

The OHIE found that Medicaid coverage significantly improves enrollees' access to medical care. Specifically, based on in-person interviews two years after the coverage lottery, the authors estimate that those enrolled in Medicaid were more likely to:

- Receive all needed care.

Medicaid coverage increased the probability that individuals reported receiving all needed medical care over the prior 12 months by 11.4 percentage points, relative to a baseline rate of 61.0 percent in the control group.[4]

- Have a usual source of clinic care.

Medicaid coverage increased the probability that individuals reported having a usual source of clinic care (e.g. a primary care physician) by 23.8 percentage points, relative to a baseline probability of 46.1 percent in the control group.[5]

- Receive recommended preventive care.

Medicaid coverage dramatically increased receipt of several important types of recommended preventive care that have been clinically demonstrated to improve health outcomes:

- Cholesterol-level screenings: Medicaid coverage increased the probability that an individual received a cholesterol-level screening in the last 12 months by 14.6 percentage points, relative to a baseline probability of 27.2 in the control group.
- Mammograms: Medicaid coverage increased the probability that women ages and 50 and older received a mammogram in the last 12 months by 29.7 percentage points, relative to a baseline probability of 28.9 percent in the control group.
- Papanicolaou tests ("pap smears"): Medicaid coverage increased the probability that a woman had received a pap smear in the last 12 months by 14.4 percentage points, relative to a baseline probability of 44.9 percent in the control group.[6]

- Receive other types of medical care.
  Medicaid coverage also increased receipt of other categories of medical care. Medicaid coverage made possible an additional 2.7 office visits over the course of a year, relative to 5.5 visits in the control group. Similarly, Medicaid increased the number of prescription medications an individual was currently taking by 0.7 prescriptions, relative to 1.8 prescriptions in the control group.

While the OHIE is uniquely well-suited to the current analysis in light of its randomized design and focus on a population that is very similar to the population that will gain coverage if more states elect to expand Medicaid, the finding that having health insurance or more generous health insurance increases access to health care services has been convincingly demonstrated in many health care settings. High-quality studies arriving at similar conclusions include the well-known RAND Health Insurance Experiment (Newhouse 1993), studies of past Medicaid expansions (e.g. Currie and Gruber 1996; Sommers, Baicker, and Epstein 2012), studies of the effect of gaining Medicare eligibility at age 65 (e.g. McWilliams et al. 2007; Card et al. 2009), and a prominent study of Massachusetts health reform (Sommers, Long, and Baicker 2014).

To translate the OHIE estimates into the number of additional individuals estimated to have specified type of health care experience in each State, the relevant point estimates were simply multiplied by the HIPSM estimates of the number of individuals who would gain coverage in that State if the State expands Medicaid coverage.[7] Several of the preventive care estimates apply only to particular age and gender subgroups; CEA estimated the share of new Medicaid enrollees who fall in the relevant subgroups using the American Community Survey and the methodology described in Appendix A and then scaled down the HIPSM estimates accordingly.

The resulting State-by-State estimates of the increase in receipt of medical care are reported in Table 2 (preventive care) and Table 3 (other utilization measures). Figure 2 summarizes the increases in utilization of preventive care that States that have not yet expanded Medicaid could achieve once expanded coverage is fully in effect, as well as the gains accruing to States that have already expanded the program. Figure 3 maps the State-level estimates of the increase in the annual number of cholesterol-level screenings if each State expands Medicaid.

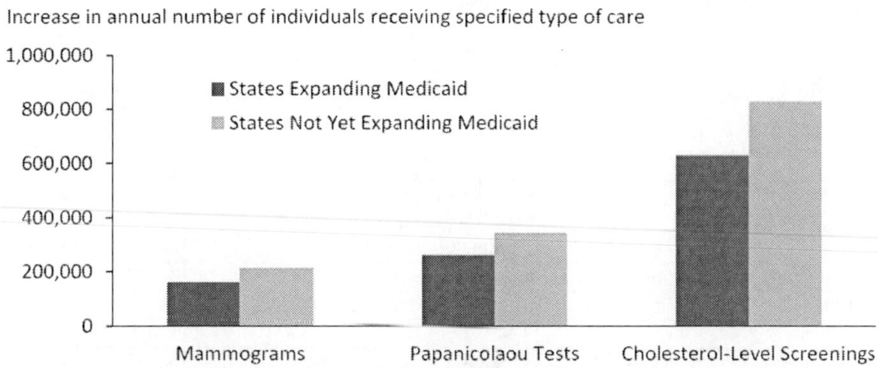

Sources: Urban Institute; Baicker et al. (2013); CEA calculations.

Note: Estimates reflect effects when expanded coverage is fully in effect. See text for methodological details. Increases in receipt of mammograms reflect only women 50 and older.

Figure 2. Projected Increase in Utilization of Preventive Care if States Expand Medicaid, by Current Expansion Status.

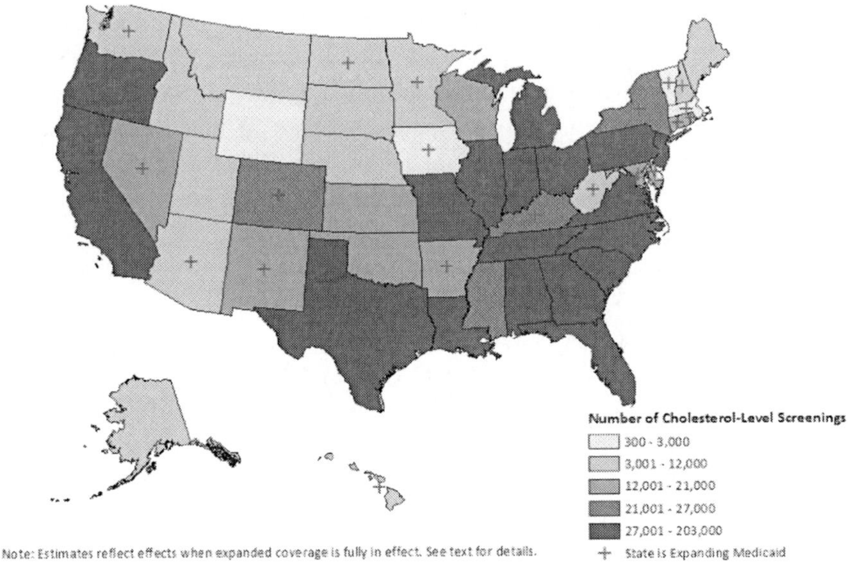

Figure 3. Projected Annual Number of Additional Cholesterol-Level Screenings if Each State Decides to Expand Medicaid.

Table 2. Number of Additional People Receiving Preventive Care if State Expands Medicaid

	Cholesterol-Level Screening in Past 12 Months	Mammogram in Past 12 Months	Papanicolaou Smear in Past 12 Months
Not Yet Expanding Medicaid	**829,300**	**214,100**	**344,900**
Alabama	34,200	9,300	14,200
Alaska	3,800	900	1,500
Florida	123,600	35,300	52,200
Georgia	69,600	17,000	28,900
Idaho	8,000	2,300	3,300
Indiana	38,200	9,000	15,200
Kansas	14,600	3,100	5,800
Louisiana	38,600	10,400	16,000
Maine	4,100	1,300	1,700
Mississippi	24,000	6,200	9,700
Missouri	36,900	9,400	14,900
Montana	5,500	1,600	2,400
Nebraska	7,000	1,600	2,900
North Carolina	54,900	13,900	23,000
Oklahoma	17,900	4,800	7,300
Pennsylvania	44,400	11,100	17,600

	Cholesterol-Level Screening in Past 12 Months	Mammogram in Past 12 Months	Papanicolaou Smear in Past 12 Months
South Carolina	28,800	8,000	12,000
South Dakota	3,800	900	1,500
Tennessee	34,100	9,500	14,000
Texas	176,000	44,100	75,200
Utah	10,800	1,900	4,500
Virginia	30,600	8,000	13,000
Wisconsin	17,500	3,800	6,700
Wyoming	2,300	700	1,100
Expanding Medicaid	**629,600**	**160,600**	**261,300**
Arizona	7,400	2,600	3,200
Arkansas	20,800	5,600	8,500
California	202,500	49,300	86,800
Colorado	22,400	5,200	9,000
Connecticut	12,200	3,100	5,100
Delaware	1,000	300	500
District of Columbia	2,800	400	1,200
Hawaii	5,700	1,600	2,300
Illinois	58,000	14,700	23,800
Iowa	2,900	600	1,200
Kentucky	25,800	6,600	10,300
Maryland	19,700	4,600	8,100
Massachusetts	300	100	100
Michigan	30,900	7,000	12,000
Minnesota	6,100	1,300	2,500
Nevada	15,300	4,300	6,500
New Hampshire	3,800	1,100	1,600
New Jersey	33,100	8,600	14,000
New Mexico	14,000	3,700	5,500
New York	24,300	8,400	10,300
North Dakota	3,100	700	1,300
Ohio	65,000	17,400	26,000
Oregon	27,100	7,100	11,300
Rhode Island	3,800	900	1,600
Vermont	600	< 100	< 100
Washington	9,300	2,200	3,900
West Virginia	11,700	3,300	4,700

Sources: Urban Institute; American Community Survey, 2010-2012; CEA calculations.

Note: Estimates reflect effects when expanded coverage is fully in effect. See text for details on the methodology. Numbers may not sum due to rounding. Mammogram estimates reflect mammograms received by women 50 and older only.

Table 3. Effects on Access to Care and Health Outcomes if State Expands Medicaid

	Additional People with a Usual Source of Clinic Care	Additional People Receiving All Needed Care in Past 12 Months	Number of Additional Physician Visits Each Year	Reduction in Number of People Experiencing Depression	Additional People Reporting Good, Very Good, or Excellent Health
Not Yet Expanding Medicaid	**1,352,000**	**651,000**	**15,368,000**	**458,000**	**757,000**
Alabama	56,000	27,000	635,000	19,000	31,000
Alaska	6,000	3,000	70,000	2,000	3,000
Florida	201,000	97,000	2,290,000	68,000	113,000
Georgia	114,000	55,000	1,291,000	38,000	64,000
Idaho	13,000	6,000	149,000	4,000	7,000
Indiana	62,000	30,000	707,000	21,000	35,000
Kansas	24,000	11,000	270,000	8,000	13,000
Louisiana	63,000	30,000	716,000	21,000	35,000
Maine	7,000	3,000	76,000	2,000	4,000
Mississippi	39,000	19,000	446,000	13,000	22,000
Missouri	60,000	29,000	683,000	20,000	34,000
Montana	9,000	4,000	103,000	3,000	5,000
Nebraska	11,000	5,000	130,000	4,000	6,000
North Carolina	90,000	43,000	1,018,000	30,000	50,000
Oklahoma	29,000	14,000	332,000	10,000	16,000
Pennsylvania	72,000	35,000	824,000	25,000	41,000
South Carolina	47,000	23,000	535,000	16,000	26,000
South Dakota	6,000	3,000	70,000	2,000	3,000
Tennessee	56,000	27,000	632,000	19,000	31,000
Texas	287,000	138,000	3,262,000	97,000	161,000
Utah	18,000	8,000	200,000	6,000	10,000
Virginia	50,000	24,000	567,000	17,000	28,000
Wisconsin	29,000	14,000	324,000	10,000	16,000
Wyoming	4,000	2,000	43,000	1,000	2,000
Expanding Medicaid	**1,026,000**	**494,000**	**11,667,000**	**348,000**	**575,000**
Arizona	12,000	6,000	138,000	4,000	7,000
Arkansas	34,000	16,000	386,000	12,000	19,000
California	330,000	159,000	3,753,000	112,000	185,000
Colorado	37,000	18,000	416,000	12,000	20,000
Connecticut	20,000	10,000	227,000	7,000	11,000
Delaware	2,000	1,000	19,000	1,000	1,000
District of Columbia	5,000	2,000	51,000	2,000	3,000
Hawaii	9,000	4,000	105,000	3,000	5,000
Illinois	95,000	45,000	1,075,000	32,000	53,000
Iowa	5,000	2,000	54,000	2,000	3,000
Kentucky	42,000	20,000	478,000	14,000	24,000

	Additional People with a Usual Source of Clinic Care	Additional People Receiving All Needed Care in Past 12 Months	Number of Additional Physician Visits Each Year	Reduction in Number of People Experiencing Depression	Additional People Reporting Good, Very Good, or Excellent Health
Maryland	32,000	15,000	365,000	11,000	18,000
Massachusetts	<1000	<1000	5,000	<1000	<1000
Michigan	50,000	24,000	572,000	17,000	28,000
Minnesota	10,000	5,000	113,000	3,000	6,000
Nevada	25,000	12,000	284,000	8,000	14,000
New Hampshire	6,000	3,000	70,000	2,000	3,000
New Jersey	54,000	26,000	613,000	18,000	30,000
New Mexico	23,000	11,000	259,000	8,000	13,000
New York	40,000	19,000	451,000	13,000	22,000
North Dakota	5,000	2,000	57,000	2,000	3,000
Ohio	106,000	51,000	1,204,000	36,000	59,000
Oregon	44,000	21,000	502,000	15,000	25,000
Rhode Island	6,000	3,000	70,000	2,000	3,000
Vermont	1,000	<1000	11,000	<1000	1,000
Washington	15,000	7,000	173,000	5,000	9,000
West Virginia	19,000	9,000	216,000	6,000	11,000

Sources: Urban Institute; American Community Survey, 2010–2012; CEA calculations.

Note: Estimates reflect effects when expanded coverage is fully in effect. See text for details on the methodology. Numbers may not sum due to rounding

Effects on Financial Security

While one important goal of the Medicaid program is to ensure that enrollees have access to medical care, an equally important goal is to protect families from large out-of-pocket medical costs and ensure that illness does not threaten families' ability to meet other important needs. To quantify the improvements in financial security resulting from State decisions to expand Medicaid under the Affordable Care Act, this analysis turns once again to the OHIE, which found that Medicaid coverage significantly improved financial security.

This analysis focuses on two specific outcomes measured in the OHIE, which were measured using in-person interviews two years after the coverage lottery:

- Catastrophic out-of-pocket costs.

Medicaid coverage nearly eliminated the risk of facing catastrophic out-of-pocket medical costs (defined in the study as out-of-pocket spending in excess of 30 percent of household income) during the prior year. Specifically, being enrolled in Medicaid reduced the probability of experiencing such an outcome by 4.5 percentage points, relative to a baseline risk of 5.5 percent in the control group.

- Trouble paying bills due to medical expenses.

  Medicaid coverage dramatically reduced the risk that an individual reported having borrowed money or skipped paying other bills due to medical expenses during the prior year. Specifically, being enrolled in Medicaid reduced the probability of experiencing such an outcome by 14.2 percentage points, relative to a baseline risk of 24.4 percent in the control group.

The OHIE also found that Medicaid coverage reduced the average amount of out-of-pocket spending and the probability of having any medical debt. In addition, in earlier work using credit report data, the OHIE investigators documented a large reduction in the probability of having had a medical bill sent to a collection agency over slightly more than one year of follow-up.

As with the health care utilization results discussed in the last subsection, the finding that health insurance improves financial security is not unique to the OHIE. Finkelstein and McKnight (2008) demonstrate that the introduction of Medicare in 1965 led to sharp reductions in seniors' exposure to large out-of-pocket medical costs. Gross and Notowidigdo (2011) examine Medicaid expansions during the 1990s and early 2000s and find that those expansions significantly reduced the risk of consumer bankruptcy.[8]

To translate the OHIE estimates into the number of individuals estimated to avoid these negative financial outcomes in each State, the OHIE point estimate was multiplied by the HIPSM estimates of the number of individuals estimated to gain coverage in that State if the State expands Medicaid coverage. The resulting State-by-State estimates of the reduction in the number of individuals facing adverse financial outcomes due to high out-of-pocket medical costs are reported in Table 4. Figure 4 summarizes the reduction in the incidence of adverse financial outcomes that States that have not yet expanded Medicaid could achieve once expanded coverage is fully in effect, as well as the gains for States that have already expanded the program. Figure 5 maps the State-level estimates of the reduction in the number of individuals borrowing money or skipping payments on other bills due to medical expenses if each State expands Medicaid.

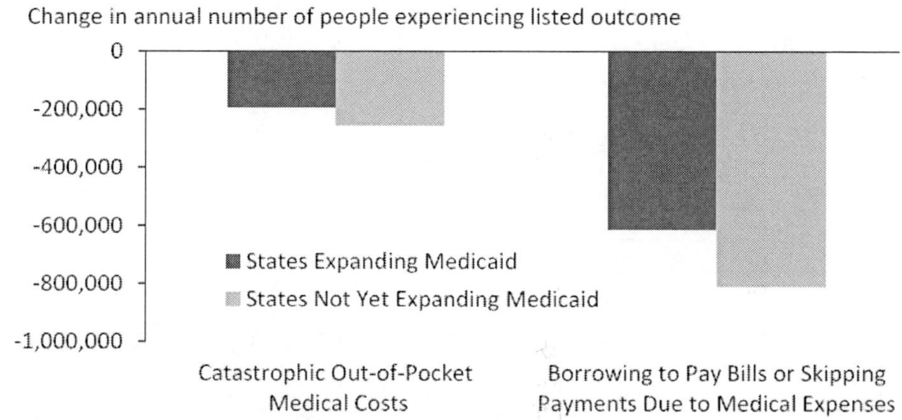

Source: Urban Institute; Baicker et al. (2013); CEA calculations.
Note: Estimates reflect effects when expanded coverage is fully in effect. See text for methodological details.

Figure 4. Projected Reduction in the Incidence of Financial Hardship if States Expand Medicaid, by Current Expansion Status.

Table 4. Reduction in Number of People Facing Financial Hardship if State Expands Medicaid

	People with Catastrophic Out-of-Pocket Costs in a Typical Year	People Borrowing to Pay Bills or Skipping Payments Due to Medical Bills
Not Yet Expanding Medicaid	**255,000**	**809,400**
Alabama	10,500	33,400
Alaska	1,200	3,700
Florida	38,000	120,600
Georgia	21,400	68,000
Idaho	2,500	7,800
Indiana	11,700	37,300
Kansas	4,500	14,200
Louisiana	11,900	37,700

Table 4. (Continued)

	People with Catastrophic Out-of-Pocket Costs in a Typical Year	People Borrowing to Pay Bills or Skipping Payments Due to Medical Bills
Maine	1,300	4,000
Mississippi	7,400	23,500
Missouri	11,300	36,000
Montana	1,700	5,400
Nebraska	2,200	6,800
North Carolina	16,900	53,600
Oklahoma	5,500	17,500
Pennsylvania	13,700	43,400
South Carolina	8,900	28,200
South Dakota	1,200	3,700
Tennessee	10,500	33,300
Texas	54,100	171,800
Utah	3,300	10,500
Virginia	9,400	29,900
Wisconsin	5,400	17,100
Wyoming	700	2,300
Expanding Medicaid	**193,600**	**614,400**
Arizona	2,300	7,300
Arkansas	6,400	20,300
California	62,300	197,700
Colorado	6,900	21,900
Connecticut	3,800	11,900
Delaware	300	1,000
District of Columbia	900	2,700
Hawaii	1,700	5,500
Illinois	17,800	56,600
Iowa	900	2,800
Kentucky	7,900	25,200
Maryland	6,000	19,200
Massachusetts	100	300
Michigan	9,500	30,100
Minnesota	1,900	6,000
Nevada	4,700	14,900
New Hampshire	1,200	3,700
New Jersey	10,200	32,300
New Mexico	4,300	13,700
New York	7,500	23,700
North Dakota	900	3,000

	People with Catastrophic Out-of-Pocket Costs in a Typical Year	People Borrowing to Pay Bills or Skipping Payments Due to Medical Bills
Ohio	20,000	63,400
Oregon	8,300	26,400
Rhode Island	1,200	3,700
Vermont	200	600
Washington	2,900	9,100
West Virginia	3,600	11,400

Sources:Urban Institute; American Community Survey, 2010-2012; CEA calculations.

Note: Estimates reflect effects when expanded coverage is fully in effect. See text for details on the methodology. Numbers may not sum due to rounding. Catastrophic medical costs defined as medical costs exceeding 30 percent of income.

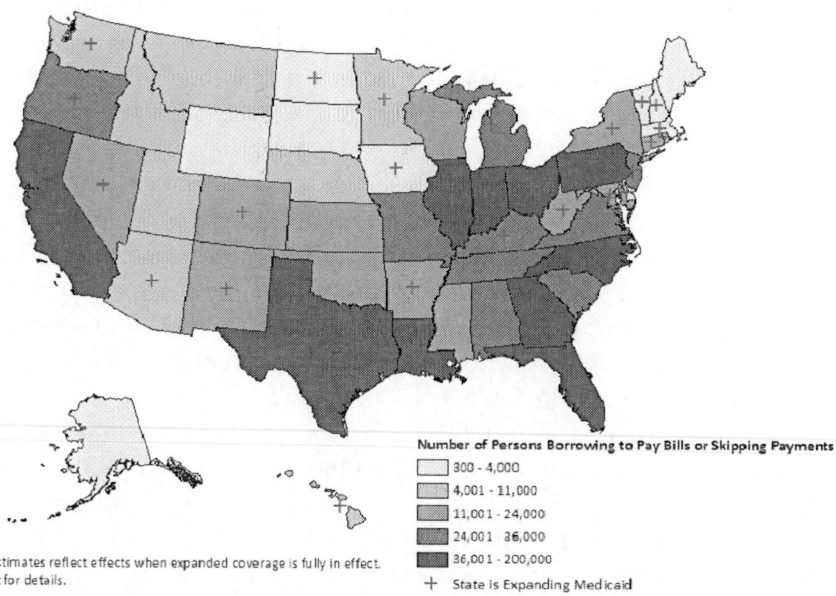

Figure 5. Projected Annual Reduction in the Number of Individuals Borrowing Money or Skipping Payments Due to Medical Expenses if Each State Decides to Expand Medicaid.

Effects on Health Outcomes

Medicaid also seeks to improve enrollees' health. The findings above showing that Medicaid increases receipt of recommended medical care—care for which there is a strong clinical evidence base demonstrating its effectiveness in improving health—justifies a strong presumption that Medicaid does indeed improve enrollees' health. Nevertheless, direct evidence that health insurance improves health is desirable.

To quantify effects on mental health, this analysis turns once more to the OHIE. The OHIE found that Medicaid coverage reduced the probability that an individual screened positive for depression on the basis of a standard eight‑question questionnaire by 9.2 percentage points, relative to a 30.0 percent baseline probability in the control group.[9] Medicaid coverage also generated improvements in self-reported mental health, as measured using a standard three-question battery on the effect of mental health on quality of life.

Two steps were used to translate OHIE's estimate that Medicaid reduced the probability of screening positive for depression into the reduction in the number of people actually experiencing depression if each State expanded Medicaid. First, the reduction in the number of people who would *screen* positive for depression was obtained by multiplying the OHIE point estimate by the HIPSM estimates of the number of individuals who will gain coverage in each State if that state expands its Medicaid program. Prior research has estimated that 88 percent of those who screen positive for depression using this screening tool are found to be experiencing major depression on the basis of a clinical interview (Kroenke et al. 2001). Thus, to obtain the final estimates of the reduction in the incidence of depression, the reduction in the number of positive screening results was multiplied by 0.88.[10] The resulting State-by-State estimates of the reduction in the number of individuals experiencing depression are reported in Table 3.

Turning to physical health, the OHIE provides clear evidence that individuals receiving Medicaid perceived themselves to be in better health. In results through approximately two years of follow-up, Medicaid coverage increased the share of individuals reporting that their health had remained the same or improved over the prior year by 7.8 percentage points, relative to a baseline probability of 80.4 percent in the control group. In earlier results through slightly more than one year of follow-up, Medicaid also increased the probability that an individual reported that his or her health was good, very good, or excellent by 13.3 percentage points, relative to a baseline probability of 54.8 percent in the control group.

To translate the OHIE estimate of the effect of Medicaid on the number of individuals reporting that they are in good, very good, or excellent health into an estimate of the number of additional people who would assess their health in this way if each State expanded Medicaid, the OHIE point estimate is simply multiplied by the number of people who will gain coverage if each

State expands its Medicaid program. The resulting State-by-State estimates are reported in Table 3 and are mapped in Figure 6. Figure 7 summarizes the improvements in this measure of health that States that have not yet expanded Medicaid could achieve once expanded coverage is fully in effect, as well as the gains for States that have already expanded the program.

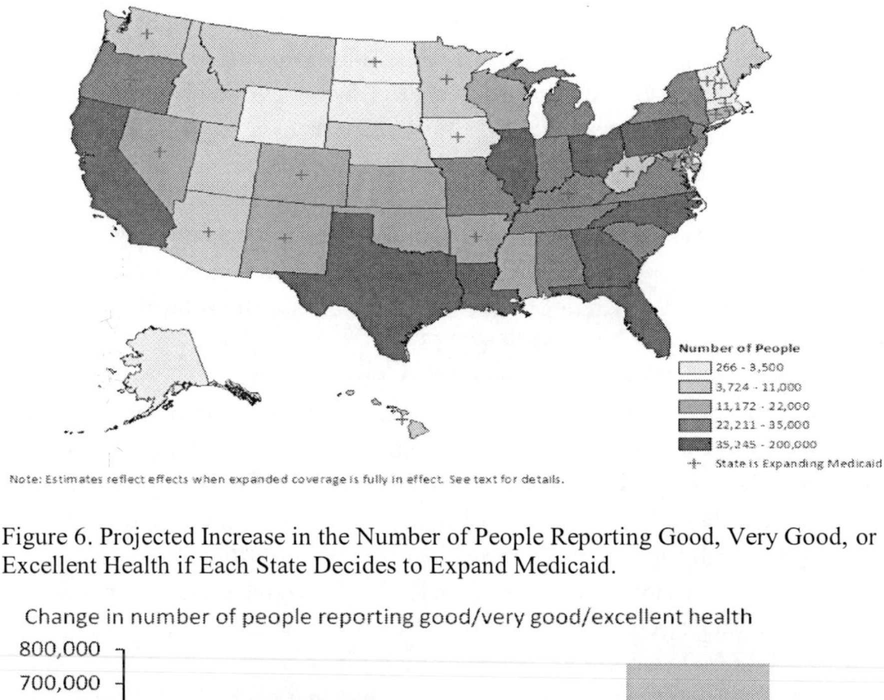

Figure 6. Projected Increase in the Number of People Reporting Good, Very Good, or Excellent Health if Each State Decides to Expand Medicaid.

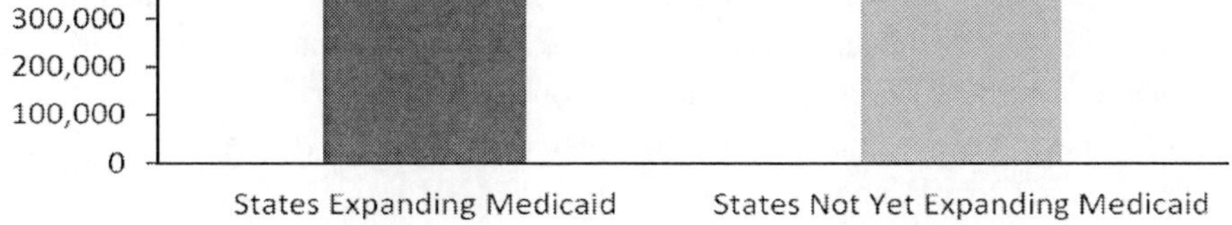

Source: Urban Institute; Finkelstein et al. (2012); CEA calculations.

Note: Estimates reflect effects when expanded coverage is fully in effect. See text for methodological details.

Figure 7. Projected Increase in Number of People Reporting Good, Very Good, or Excellent Health if States Expand Medicaid, by Current Expansion Status.

The limited sample size of the OHIE makes it more difficult to reach firm conclusions about the effect of Medicaid on objective measures of physical health since the OHIE estimates were generally imprecise. The OHIE did attempt to measure the effect of Medicaid coverage on several physical health outcomes, including the incidence of high blood pressure, high cholesterol, and poor control of blood sugar. The study's *point estimates* (roughly speaking, a point estimate is the most likely single value in light of a study's data) showed some improvement in each of these domains. For example, the study's point estimate was that Medicaid reduced the incidence of elevated blood pressure by 1.3 percentage points, relative to a baseline incidence of 16.3 percent in the control group; the point estimates for the other measured dimensions of physical health were, in proportional terms, similar or larger. In early results, the OHIE also reported a point estimate suggesting that Medicaid reduced mortality over a follow-up period of slightly more than one year. These point estimates would generally be clinically meaningful if they exactly reflected reality (Frakt 2013a; Frakt 2013b).

However, the OHIE's sample size was (by necessity) quite limited, so the precision with which these changes in health outcomes could be measured was also limited. As a result, these estimated improvements in physical health fell far short of statistical significance, and it is impossible to determine with any confidence whether the point estimates described above arose because Medicaid actually generated improvements in physical health or if Medicaid actually has negligible effects on physical health, and these estimates were simply obtained by chance. For example, while the study's point estimate was that Medicaid reduced the incidence of high blood pressure by 1.3 percentage points, a 95 percent confidence interval around that estimate stretches from a 7.2 percentage point reduction in incidence to a 4.5 percentage point increase in incidence. Closely related, it may not have been reasonable to expect the OHIE to find statistically significant improvements in physical health stemming from Medicaid coverage. To be reliably detected by the OHIE, the effects of Medicaid on physical health would have had to be quite large, often larger than what seems medically plausible (Frakt 2013a; Frakt 2013b; Richardson, Carroll, and Frakt 2013; Mulligan 2013).

In light of the limitations of the OHIE for learning about the effects of Medicaid on objective physical health outcomes, it is useful to examine a parallel literature that uses "quasi- experiments" created by past policy changes to study how Medicaid coverage affects health outcomes. The disadvantage of relying on quasi-experimental research is that it is more vulnerable to unobserved confounding factors than research using a randomized research design. However, these quasi‑experimental studies have the important advantage that they can often draw on much larger samples and, thus, deliver much more precise estimates.

Two recent quasi‑experimental studies are particularly relevant in this context since they examine insurance expansions that, like State Medicaid expansions under the Affordable Care Act, primarily affect low‑ or moderate‑income adults. Sommers, Long, and Baicker (2014) study the mortality effects of Massachusetts health reform, which primarily affected adults with incomes similar to or modestly higher than those affected by the Affordable Care Act's Medicaid expansion, by comparing mortality trends in Massachusetts counties to mortality trends in demographically similar counties in the rest of the country. They find that the mortality rate for Massachusetts adults fell by 2.9 percent from the years before reform to the years after reform, relative to the comparison counties. The authors document that mortality followed similar trends in Massachusetts counties and comparison counties before reform, that the mortality gains were concentrated in counties with lower incomes and lower insurance coverage rates prior to reform, and that the improvements were primarily in causes of death believed to be avoidable with better health care; all of these findings are consistent with the interpretation that the observed fall in mortality in Massachusetts was caused by the expansion of insurance coverage. Notably, the authors' estimate falls well within the very wide 95 percent confidence interval associated with the imprecise corresponding OHIE estimate.

Sommers, Baicker, and Epstein (2012) examine pre-ACA expansions of Medicaid coverage to low-income adults in Arizona, New York, and Maine. Much like Sommers, Long, and Baicker, the authors estimate how these Medicaid expansions affected the risk of death by comparing mortality trends in the three expansion states to mortality trends in neighboring states. They find that the mortality rate for adults fell by 6.1 percent in the expansion states relative to non-expanding States in the years around the reform. They document that mortality trends were similar in expansion and non-expansion states before reform and that the mortality gains were concentrated in lower-income counties, consistent with the interpretation that the fall in mortality in the expansion states was caused by expanded insurance coverage. This estimate is also not statistically different from the imprecise corresponding OHIE estimate.

These are not the only quasi-experimental studies examining the link between health insurance status and health outcomes, although they are the two that are most relevant to evaluating the consequences of States' Medicaid expansion decisions. Currie and Gruber (1994), Currie and Gruber (1996), Meyer and Wherry (2012) examine past Medicaid expansions affecting pregnant women, children, and teens, respectively, and find that those coverage expansions reduced mortality. Card, Dobkin, and Maestas (2009) document a discrete reduction in mortality for patients arriving at the hospital with "non-deferrable" conditions at age 65, coinciding with the beginning of eligibility for Medicare. Levy and Meltzer (2008) undertake a careful review of the quasi-experimental literature and conclude that, while that literature is not unanimous on this question, the balance of the evidence demonstrates that expanding access to health insurance coverage improves health for specific well-studied populations. The results from Sommers, Long, and Baicker (2014) and Sommers, Baicker, and Epstein (2012) provide strong evidence that this general conclusion that expanded coverage improves health applies to coverage expansions that affect low- and moderate-income adults, like Medicaid expansions under the Affordable Care Act.

Effects on State Economies and the National Economy

In addition to their effects on insurance coverage, access to health care, and health and wellbeing, States decisions to expand Medicaid will also have immediate macroeconomic benefits by drawing additional Federal funding into State economies. As described in greater detail below, this additional Federal funding will increase demand for both medical and non-medical goods and services. Over the next few years, while the recovery from the 2007-2009 recession remains incomplete and slack remains in the economy, this increase in demand will boost overall employment and economic activity.

In detail, when a State elects to expand its Medicaid program, the Federal government finances additional payments to medical providers in the State in exchange for providing medical services to the new Medicaid enrollees. These additional Medicaid outlays are only partially offset by reduced Federal spending on premium tax credits and cost-sharing assistance for individuals in that State with incomes between 100 and 138 percent of the FPL who switch from receiving coverage through the Marketplaces to receiving coverage through Medicaid.

CEA has used data from the Congressional Budget Office and Urban Institute data to estimate the additional Federal outlays each State would have triggered if it had expanded Medicaid by January 1, 2014; the detailed methodology is presented in Appendix B. On the basis of this methodology,

CEA estimates that if the 24 States that have not yet expanded Medicaid had done so as of January 1, 2014, that would have triggered an increase in Federal outlays in those States totaling $88 billion during calendar years 2014 through 2016. States that have already expanded Medicaid will generate additional Federal outlays of $84 billion during this period. State-by-State estimates of the additional Federal outlays resulting from each State's decision to expand Medicaid are reported in Table 5.[11]

In order to quantify the effects of these additional Federal outlays on States' economies and the economy of the Nation as a whole, CEA has undertaken a standard "fiscal multiplier" analysis. In brief, when the government purchases additional goods and services, that spurs hiring and purchases of investment goods and raw materials to produce those goods and services. As those newly-hired workers and producers spend the income they have earned, they spur additional hiring and purchases, which in turn sets off yet another round of increases in spending, and so on. Economists summarize this sequence of macroeconomic effects via a "fiscal multiplier," which measures the total number of dollars of additional economic activity arising from a one-dollar fiscal change. The 2014 *Economic Report of the President* provides a detailed discussion of the theoretical basis for this type of analysis and the empirical literature underlying CEA's estimates of the multiplier for different types of fiscal changes (CEA 2014). As described therein, CEA's multiplier estimates fall well within the range of estimates used by other analysts, including the Congressional Budget Office.

The appropriate multiplier to use for evaluating the macroeconomic consequences of States' Medicaid expansion decisions depends on how the additional Federal outlays triggered by States' decisions enter State economies. In practice, these outlays will take three main paths:

- Additional utilization of medical care.

Consistent with the evidence described earlier in this report, much of the additional Federal funding will fund additional medical care for newly enrolled Medicaid enrollees, increasing overall demand for medical goods and services. For dollars entering the economy this way, CEA uses a GDP multiplier of 1.5, consistent with CEA's estimate of the multiplier for direct government spending.

- Lower out-of-pocket medical costs.

Also consistent with the evidence presented earlier in this report, some of the additional Federal funding will protect enrollees from high out-of-pocket medical costs, permitting families to redirect dollars to other pressing needs and boosting demand for a wide variety of goods and services.[12] For dollars entering the economy this way, CEA uses a GDP multiplier of 1.5, consistent with CEA's estimate of the multiplier for payments to low-income households.

- Reductions in uncompensated care.

The remainder of the additional Federal funding will compensate providers for the cost of providing care that previously went unreimbursed. In turn, those funds will flow through to the entities that were previously bearing the cost of that uncompensated care, some combination of State and local governments, privately-insured individuals, and medical providers.[13] Those additional funds will permit those entities to increase their demand for goods and services (or, in the case of governments, reduce taxes on households, increasing households' demand for goods and services).
For reductions in uncompensated care costs borne by State and local governments, CEA uses a multiplier of 1.1, consistent with CEA's estimate of the multiplier for payments to State and local governments. For other reductions in uncompensated care costs, CEA uses a GDP multiplier of 0.8, consistent with CEA's estimate of the multiplier applicable to individual tax cuts.

Based on recent estimates of per capita uncompensated care costs among the uninsured (Coughlin et al., 2013), a reasonable estimate is that around 30 percent of the additional Medicaid spending will defray uncompensated care costs.[14] While, in practice, State and local governments are likely to realize a significant fraction of these savings, in the interest of being conservative, CEA has assumed that these savings accrue entirely to providers and other payers, which leads to a composite multiplier of 1.29 for each additional dollar of Federal outlays resulting from a State's decision to expand Medicaid. The magnitude of this composite multiplier is not particularly sensitive to alternative assumptions about the extent to which expanding Medicaid defrays uncompensated care costs versus entering the economy through other channels. To generate estimates of the macroeconomic effect of State Medicaid expansion decisions, the estimated fiscal effects of State decisions to expand Medicaid and the multiplier estimates described above were used as inputs into the CEA multiplier model, which has been described in previous CEA publications (CEA 2014). The CEA model then produces quarterly estimates of the effect of States' decisions about whether to expand Medicaid on employment and overall economic activity.[15]

The estimates generated by the CEA multiplier model assume that, as is the case now, there is slack in the economy and productive resources are not fully employed.[16] When the economy returns to full employment, these demand-side effects will become much smaller and eventually disappear entirely because an increase in labor demand in one sector will mostly tend to reallocate workers away from other sectors. Looking forward, the Federal Reserve and many private forecasters expect the economy to remain short of full employment until late 2016. For the purposes of this analysis, the CEA assumes that Federal outlays spurred by States' Medicaid expansion decisions will have their full macroeconomic effects through the middle of 2015 and that these effects phase down gradually thereafter, reaching zero by the beginning of 2017. While this approach is somewhat ad hoc, it likely provides a reasonable approximation of the actual effects.

State-by-State estimates of the effect on employment and total output if each State decides to expand Medicaid are reported in Tables 5 and 6. Figure 8 summarizes the number of jobs that States that have not yet expanded Medicaid could have created if they had expanded the program as of January 1, 2014, as well as the gains that will be achieved by States that have already expanded the program. Figure 9 maps the cumulative job-years from 2014 through 2017 that would have been created if each State had expanded Medicaid as of January 1, 2014.

While this subsection focuses on the short-run macroeconomic benefits of expanded insurance coverage, States' decisions to expand Medicaid could affect employment and economic activity over the longer run as well. Healthier workers who are less financially stressed and in better mental health may be more able to effectively participate in the labor force and have higher productivity on the job. On the other hand, access to coverage through Medicaid would likely cause some workers to reduce their labor supply, either because having Medicaid coverage eliminate the need to work in order to obtain health insurance or because Medicaid causes individuals to choose to work less in order to avoid losing access to Medicaid coverage.[17] Reductions in labor supply of the latter kind generally reduce economic efficiency. In contrast, reductions in labor supply of the former kind can improve economic efficiency if they permit workers to choose to pursue a higher-value alternative activity like caring for children or other family members, pursuing additional education, or starting a business; some reductions in this category are commonly described as reflecting reductions in "job" or "employment lock."

The evidence on the net effects of Medicaid on labor supply for populations like those affected the Affordable Care Act's Medicaid expansion is mixed. The highest-quality evidence comes from the OHIE, which concluded that Medicaid enrollment had small and statistically insignificant effects on labor supply (Baicker et al. 2013b). Some non-randomized quasi-experimental studies have, however, found that Medicaid causes statistically significant reductions in labor supply. Dague, DeLeire, and Leininger (2014) study an episode in which a portion of Wisconsin's Medicaid program was closed to new enrollment and conclude that Medicaid enrollment drove modest reductions in labor supply. Garthwaite, Gross, and Notowidigdo (2014) study a large-scale disenrollment from Tennessee's TennCare program in the mid-2000s and estimate much larger effects on labor supply. It is generally not clear what portions of these labor supply responses occur through channels that increase, reduce, or do not affect economic efficiency.

The reasons why different studies have reached widely differing conclusions about the effect of Medicaid on labor supply is not well understood. The differences could reflect differences in the populations affected by these different policy changes or the time period during which those changes occurred. Notably, the population studied by Garthwaite, Gross, and Notowidigdo is somewhat higher income than the population affected by the Affordable Care Act's Medicaid expansion. Another possibility is that the differences reflect statistical sampling errors; because none of the studies are able to measure effects on labor supply with absolute precision (with the Garthwaite, Gross, and Notowidigdo study being particularly imprecise), it would not be surprising to see some dispersion in these estimates even if all the studies are measuring the same underlying response. Finally, the differences could arise because the quasi-experimental estimates are contaminated by unobserved differences between those who do and do not enroll in Medicaid that the authors are unable to fully control for, in which case the experimental result from the OHIE would provide the only reliable estimate. In any case, labor supply responses are not likely to be particularly relevant to macroeconomic outcomes during the period examined in this report. As long as slack remains in the labor market and there are more workers seeking work than there are available job openings, a worker who reduces his labor supply due to the availability of Medicaid coverage will often simply be replaced by another job-seeker (CBO 2014a). Thus, any labor supply effects that do exist are likely to be substantially attenuated for the next few years.

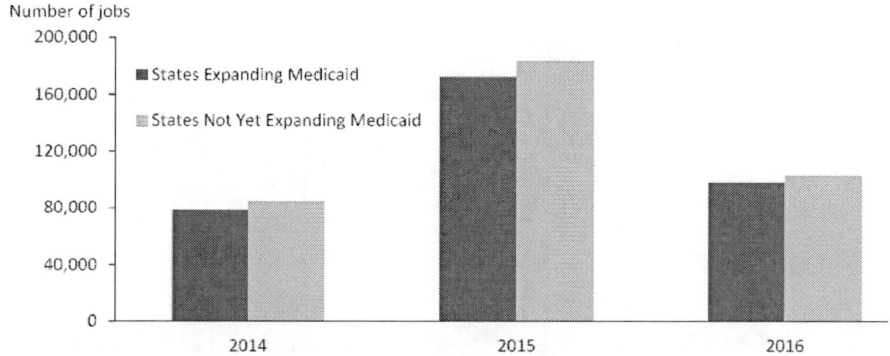

Source: Congressional Budget Office; Urban Institute; CEA calculations.

Figure 8. Projected Increase in Employment if States Expand Medicaid, by Current Expansion Status.

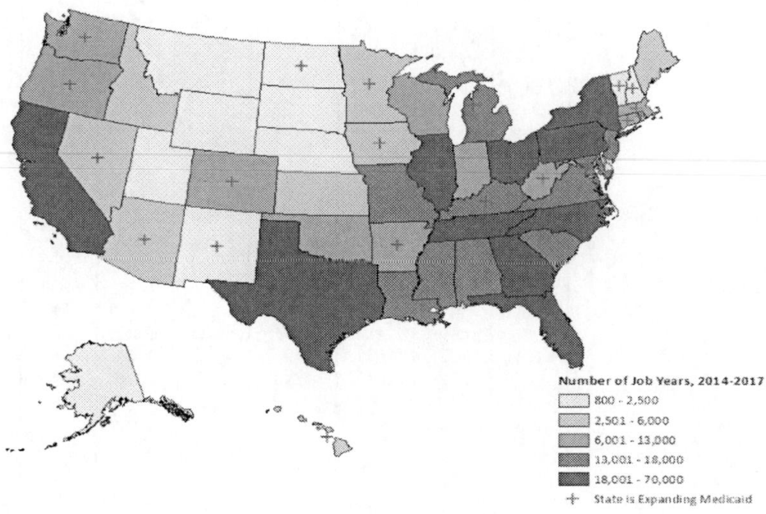

Figure 9. Projected Number of Additional Job Years from 2014-2017 if Each State Had Decided to Expand Medicaid as of January 1, 2014.

Table 5. Increase in Federal Spending and Employment if State Expands Medicaid

	Net Increase in Federal Spending (Millions of Dollars; Calendar Years)				Increase in Employment (Number of Workers; Calendar Years)			
	2014	2015	2016	Cumulative, 2014-2016	2014	2015	2016	Cumulative Job Years, 2014-2017
Not Yet Expanding Medicaid	**26,480**	**29,760**	**31,870**	**88,110**	**84,800**	**183,800**	**103,100**	**378,700**
Alabama	1,020	1,220	1,390	3,630	3,200	7,300	4,300	15,100
Alaska	100	110	120	330	300	700	400	1,400
Florida	4,410	5,060	5,530	15,010	14,100	30,900	17,600	63,800
Georgia	2,270	2,620	2,880	7,770	7,200	15,900	9,100	32,900
Idaho	200	210	210	620	600	1,300	700	2,700
Indiana	950	940	860	2,760	3,100	6,300	3,100	12,800
Kansas	290	280	250	820	1,000	1,900	900	3,800
Louisiana	1,010	1,120	1,200	3,330	3,200	7,000	3,900	14,400
Maine	210	240	260	710	700	1,500	800	3,000
Mississippi	1,020	1,210	1,370	3,600	3,200	7,200	4,300	15,000
Missouri	1,170	1,330	1,440	3,950	3,700	8,200	4,600	16,900
Montana	120	120	110	350	400	800	400	1,600
Nebraska	160	160	140	460	500	1,100	500	2,200
North Carolina	2,740	3,220	3,600	9,560	8,700	19,400	11,300	40,200
Oklahoma	520	560	570	1,650	1,700	3,500	1,900	7,300
Pennsylvania	2,460	2,770	2,970	8,200	7,900	17,100	9,600	35,200
South Carolina	1,030	1,160	1,250	3,450	3,300	7,200	4,000	14,800
South Dakota	130	140	150	420	400	900	500	1,900
Tennessee	1,500	1,730	1,900	5,130	4,800	10,500	6,000	21,700
Texas	4,180	4,640	4,910	13,730	13,400	28,800	16,000	59,400
Utah	200	120	<10	310	700	1,100	300	2,100
Virginia	940	1,050	1,110	3,090	3,000	6,500	3,600	13,300
Wisconsin	790	870	920	2,580	2,500	5,500	3,000	11,200
Wyoming	80	90	100	270	300	600	300	1,200
Expanding Medicaid	**24,680**	**28,200**	**30,740**	**83,620**	**78,600**	**172,400**	**98,200**	**356,100**
Arizona	430	280	60	760	1,500	2,400	700	4,700
Arkansas	810	910	980	2,690	2,600	5,600	3,200	11,500
California	4,740	5,530	6,160	16,430	15,000	33,400	19,400	69,100
Colorado	680	780	850	2,310	2,200	4,800	2,700	9,900
Connecticut	530	590	630	1,760	1,700	3,700	2,100	7,600
Delaware	120	130	150	400	400	800	500	1,700
District of Columbia	50	60	60	180	200	400	200	800
Hawaii	210	240	260	710	700	1,500	800	3,000
Illinois	1,430	1,610	1,730	4,770	4,600	9,900	5,600	20,500
Iowa	200	180	150	530	700	1,300	600	2,600
Kentucky	1,220	1,430	1,590	4,240	3,900	8,600	5,000	17,800
Maryland	980	1,230	1,470	3,680	3,000	7,100	4,400	14,900
Massachusetts	460	550	630	1,640	1,400	3,300	1,900	6,800
Michigan	1,120	1,250	1,340	3,710	3,600	7,800	4,300	16,000
Minnesota	300	290	250	840	1,000	2,000	900	4,000

	Net Increase in Federal Spending (Millions of Dollars; Calendar Years)				Increase in Employment (Number of Workers; Calendar Years)			
	2014	2015	2016	Cumulative, 2014-2016	2014	2015	2016	Cumulative Job Years, 2014-2017
New Hampshire	160	180	190	530	500	1,100	600	2,300
New Jersey	1,140	1,380	1,590	4,110	3,600	8,200	4,900	17,000
New Mexico	190	110	<10	290	700	1,000	300	2,000
New York	3,650	4,340	4,920	12,910	11,500	25,900	15,300	53,800
North Dakota	160	190	220	580	500	1,200	700	2,400
Ohio	3,690	4,330	4,860	12,870	11,700	26,100	15,200	54,000
Oregon	620	540	390	1,550	2,100	3,900	1,700	7,800
Rhode Island	200	240	260	700	600	1,400	800	2,900
Vermont	70	90	110	280	200	500	300	1,100
Washington	510	530	530	1,570	1,600	3,400	1,800	7,000
West Virginia	620	730	830	2,180	1,900	4,400	2,600	9,100

Sources: Urban Institute; Congressional Budget Office; CEA calculations.
Notes: See text for details on the methodology. Numbers may not sum due to rounding.

Table 6. Increase in Gross Domestic Product if State Expands Medicaid

	Additional GDP (Millions of Dollars; Calendar Years)			
	2014	2015	2016	Cumulative, 2014–2017
Not Yet Expanding Medicaid	**19,610**	**32,150**	**14,670**	**66,440**
Alabama	740	1,280	620	2,650
Alaska	70	120	60	250
Florida	3,250	5,420	2,520	11,190
Georgia	1,670	2,790	1,310	5,770
Idaho	150	230	100	480
Indiana	730	1,080	430	2,240
Kansas	220	320	130	670
Louisiana	750	1,220	550	2,520
Maine	150	260	120	530
Mississippi	740	1,280	620	2,640
Missouri	870	1,430	660	2,960
Montana	90	140	60	280
Nebraska	130	180	70	380
North Carolina	2,010	3,410	1,630	7,040
Oklahoma	390	620	270	1,280
Pennsylvania	1,820	2,990	1,370	6,180
South Carolina	760	1,250	580	2,590
South Dakota	100	160	70	330
Tennessee	1,100	1,850	870	3,810
Texas	3,100	5,040	2,270	10,420
Utah	170	180	30	370
Virginia	690	1,130	510	2,340

Table 6. (Continued)

	Additional GDP (Millions of Dollars; Calendar Years)			
	2014	2015	2016	Cumulative, 2014–2017
Wisconsin	590	950	430	1,970
Wyoming	60	100	40	210
Expanding Medicaid	**18,200**	**30,240**	**14,040**	**62,470**
Arizona	350	400	80	830
Arkansas	600	980	450	2,020
California	3,470	5,870	2,790	12,130
Colorado	500	840	390	1,730
Connecticut	390	640	290	1,330
Delaware	90	140	70	300
District of Columbia	40	70	30	140
Hawaii	160	260	120	530
Illinois	1,060	1,740	800	3,590
Iowa	160	220	80	450
Kentucky	890	1,510	720	3,120
Maryland	700	1,270	650	2,610
Massachusetts	340	580	280	1,190
Michigan	830	1,360	620	2,800
Minnesota	230	340	130	690
Nevada	290	500	240	1,040
New Hampshire	120	190	90	400
New Jersey	830	1,440	710	2,980
New Mexico	150	170	20	340
New York	2,660	4,570	2,210	9,440
North Dakota	120	200	100	420
Ohio	2,700	4,590	2,190	9,470
Oregon	490	660	220	1,360
Rhode Island	150	250	120	520
Vermont	50	100	50	200
Washington	380	590	250	1,230
West Virginia	450	770	370	1,590

Sources: Urban Institute; Congressional Budget Office; CEA calculations.
Notes: See text for details on the methodology. Numbers may not sum due to rounding.

This report documents the far-reaching benefits that States that have already expanded Medicaid under the Affordable Care Act will receive, and the benefits that States that have not yet expanded the program could achieve if they elected to do so. In particular, this analysis shows that by expanding their Medicaid programs, States can improve access to essential medical care, reduce financial hardship, improve their citizens' mental health and well-being, and claim billions of dollars in Federal funding that could boost their economies today. The Administration hopes that more States will decide to take advantage of these opportunities in the months and years ahead and stands ready to work with States to make these opportunities a reality.

REFERENCES

Baicker, Katherine, et al. 2013. "The Oregon Experiment – Medicaid's Effects on Clinical Outcomes." *New England Journal of Medicine* 368, no. 18: 1713–1722.

_____. 2013. "The Impact of Medicaid on Labor Force Activity and Program Participation: Evidence from the Oregon Health Insurance Experiment." Working Paper 19547. Cambridge, MA: National Bureau of Economic Research.

Card, David, Carlos Dobkin, Nicole Maestas. 2009. "Does Medicare Save Lives?" *The Quarterly Journal of Economics* 124, no 2: 597–636.

(CBO) Congressional Budget Office. 2012a. "Estimates for the Insurance Coverage Provisions of the Affordable Care Act Updated for the Recent Supreme Court Decision." http://www.cbo.gov/publication/43472.

_____. 2012b. "Updated Budget Projections: Fiscal Years 2012 to 2022." http://www.cbo.gov/publication/43119.

_____. 2014a. "The Budget and Economic Outlook: 2014 to 2024." http://www.cbo.gov/publication/45010.

_____. 2014b. "Updated Estimates of the Effects of the Insurance Coverage Provisions of the Affordable Care Act, April 2014." http://www.cbo.gov/publication/45231.

(CEA) Council of Economic Advisers. 2014. "Economic Report of the President."

(CMS) Centers for Medicare and Medicaid Services. 2014. "Medicaid & CHIP: April 2014 Monthly Applications, Eligibility Determinations, and Enrollment Report." http://www.medicaid.gov/AffordableCareAct/Medicaid-Moving-Forward-2014/Downloads/April-2014-Enrollment-Report.pdf.

Cohen Ross, Donna, et al. 2009. "A Foundation for Health Reform: Findings of a 50 State Survey of Eligibility Rules, Enrollment and Renewal Procedures, and Cost-Sharing Practices in Medicaid and CHIP for

Children and Parents During 2009, Data Tables." http://kaiserfamilyfoundation.files.wordpress.com/2013/01/8028_t.pdf.

Coughlin, Teresa A., et al. 2014. "An Estimated $84.9 Billion in Uncompensated Care Was Provided in 2013; ACA Payment Cuts Could Challenge Providers." *Health Affairs* 33, no 5: 807814.

Currie, Janet and Jonathan Gruber. 1996. "Health Insurance Eligibility, Utilization of Medical Care, and Child Health." *The Quarterly Journal of Economics* 111, no 2: 431466.

_____. 1994. "Saving Babies: The Efficacy and Cost of Recent Changes in the Medicaid Eligibility of Pregnant Women." *The Journal of Political Economy* 104, no 6: 12631296.

Dague, Laura, and Thomas DeLeire, and Lindsey Leininger. 2014. "The Effect of Public Insurance Coverage for Childless Adults on Labor Supply." Working Paper 20111. Cambridge, MA: National Bureau of Economic Research.

Eibner, Christine, et al. 2010. "Establishing State Health Insurance Exchanges: Implications for Health Insurance Enrollment, Spending, and Small Businesses."
http://www.rand.org/content/dam/rand/pubs/technical_reports/2010/RAND_TR825.p df.

Finkelstein, Amy and Robin McKnight. 2008. "What did Medicare Do? The Initial Impact of Medicare on Mortality and Out of Pocket Medical Spending." *Journal of Public Economics* 92, no. 7: 1644-1668.

Finkelstein, Amy, et al. 2012. "The Oregon Health Insurance Experiment: Evidence from the First Year." *The Quarterly Journal of Economics* 127, no 3: 1057-1106.

Frakt, Austin. 2013a. "My Reply to Jim Manzi." http://theincidentaleconomist.com/wordpress/my-reply-to-jim-manzi/.

_____.. 2013b. "The Oregon Medicaid Study and Cholesterol."
http://theincidentaleconomist.com/wordpress/the-oregon-medicaid-study-andcholesterol/.

Garthwaite, Craig, Tal Gross, and Matthew Notowidigdo. 2014. "Public Health Insurance, Labor Supply, and Employment Lock." *Quarterly Journal of Economics* 129, no. 2: 653-696.

Gruber, Jonathan and Aaron Yelowitz. 1999. "Public Health Insurance and Private Savings." *Journal of Political Economy* 107, no. 6: 1249-1274.

Guttmacher Institute. 2014. "Medicaid Family Planning Eligibility Expansions."
http://www.guttmacher.org/statecenter/spibs/spib_SMFPE.pdf.

Gross, Tal and Matthew J. Notowidigdo. 2011. "Health insurance and the consumer bankruptcy decision: Evidence from expansions of Medicaid." *Journal of Public Economics* 95, no 7-8: 767-778.

Heberlein, Martha et al. 2013. "Getting into Gear for 2014: Findings from a 50-State Survey of Eligibility, Enrollment, Renewal, and Cost-sharing Policies in Medicaid and CHIP, 2012- 2013." http://kaiserfamily foundation.files.wordpress.com/2013/05/8401.pdf.

Holahan, John, Matthew Buettgens, Stan Dorn. 2013. "The Cost of Not Expanding Medicaid." http://kaiserfamilyfoundation.files.wordpress.com /2013/07/8457-the-cost-

Holahan, John, et al. 2012. "The Cost and Coverage Implications of the ACA Medicaid Expansion: National and State-by-State Analysis." http://kaiserfamilyfoundation.files.wordpress.com/2013/01/8384.pdf.

Huang, Elbert S. and Kenneth Finegold. 2013. "Seven Million Americans Live in Areas Where Demand for Primary Care May Exceed Supply by More than 10 Percent." *Health Affairs* 32, no. 3: 614-621.

(KFF) Kaiser Family Foundation. 2009. "Expanding Health Coverage for Low-Income Adults: Filling the Gaps in Medicaid Eligibility."

_____.http://kaiserfamilyfoundation.files.wordpress.com/2013/01/7900.pdf.

.2010. "Expanding Medicaid to Low-Income Childless Adults Under Health Reform: Key Lessons from State Experiences." http://kaiserfamilyfoundation.files.wordpress.com/2013/01/8087.pdf.

Kenney, Genevieve M., et al. 2012. "Opting in to the Medicaid Expansion under the ACA: Who Are the Uninsured Adults Who Could Gain Coverage?" http://www.urban

Kroenke, Kurt, Robert L. Spitzer, Janet B.W. Williams. 2001. "The PHQ-9: Validity of a Brief Depression Severity Measure." *Journal of General Internal Medicine* 16, no. 9: 606-613.

Levy, Helen and David Meltzer. 2008. "The Impact of Health Insurance on Health." *Annual Review of Public Health* 29, 399-409.

Long, Sharon K. et al. 2014. "Early Estimates Indicate Rapid Increase in Health Insurance Coverage under the ACA: A Promising Start." http://hrms.urban

McWilliams, Michael J. et al. 2007. "Use of Health Services by Previously Uninsured Medicare Beneficiaries." *New England Journal of Medicine* 357, no. 2: 143-153.

Meyer, Bruce D. and Wherry, Laura R. "Saving Teens: Using a Policy Discontinuity to Estimate the Effects of Medicaid Eligibility." Working Paper 18309. Cambridge, MA: National Bureau of Economic Research.

Mulligan, Casey B. 2013. "The Perils of Significant Misunderstandings in Evaluating Medicaid." *The New York Times*. http://mobile.nytimes.com/blogs/

Newhouse, Joseph P. 1993. *Free for All? Lessons from the RAND Health Insurance Experiment*. Harvard University Press.

Richardson, Sam, Aaron Carroll, Austin Frakt. 2013. "More Medicaid Study Power Calculations." http://theincidentaleconomist.com/wordpress/more-medicaid-study-powercalculations-our-rejected-nejm-letter/.

Ruggles, Steven, et al. 2010. "Integrated Public Use Microdata Series: Version 5.0 [Machine-readable database]." Minneapolis: University of Minnesota.

Sommers, Benjamin D., Katherine Baicker, and Arnold M. Epstein. 2012. "Mortality and Access to Care among Adults after State Medicaid Expansions." *The New England Journal of Medicine* 367, no. 11: 1025-1034.

Sommers, Benjamin D., Sharon K. Long, and Katherine Baicker. 2014. "Changes in Mortality after Massachusetts Health Care Reform: A Quasi-Experimental Study." *Annals of Internal Medicine* 160, no. 9: 585-593.

Sonfield, Adam, Casey Alrich, and Rachel Benson Gold. 2008. "State Government Innovation in the Design and Implementation of Medicaid Family Planning Expansions." http://www.guttmacher.org/pubs/2008/03/28/StateMFPEpractices.pdf.

Taubman, Sarah L., et al. 2014. "Medicaid Increases Emergency-Department Use: Evidence from Oregon's Health Insurance Experiment." *Science* 343: 263-268.

Witters, Dan. 2014. "Uninsured Rate Drops More in States Embracing Health Law: Medicaid Expansion, State Exchanges Linked to Faster Reduction in Uninsured Rate." http://www.gallup.com/poll/-168539/uninsured-

Appendix A: Estimating the Age and Gender Mix of Individuals Who Would Gain Coverage if Their State Expands Medicaid

Several of the OHIE estimates of the effect of Medicaid on receipt of preventive care apply only to particular age or gender subgroups. Unfortunately, the published HIPSM estimates of the increase in insurance coverage arising from States' decisions to expand Medicaid do not detail the ages and genders of the individuals who would gain coverage. To address this issue, CEA estimated the share of new Medicaid enrollees who fall in the relevant subgroups using the Census Bureau's American Community Survey (ACS), a large household survey that collects information on income, insurance status, state of residence, and other relevant family characteristics.[18]

In detail, this was done in two steps. First, CEA identified individuals likely to gain coverage through Medicaid if their State expanded the program using the following criteria; namely, individuals who: (1) are adults age 19 to 64 with family income under 138 percent of the FPL; (2) were not eligible for Medicaid under pre-ACA State Medicaid income eligibility criteria;[19] (3) do not report being enrolled in Medicaid;[20] and (4) do not report being enrolled in employer-sponsored coverage. Among that group, it is straightforward to estimate the share of potential new enrollees falling in each age-gender subgroup of interest. These shares can then be applied to the State-level HIPSM estimates to obtain the increase in insurance in each relevant age-gender subgroup as a result of each State's decision to expand Medicaid.

In implementing this approach, income is defined as total cash income minus Supplemental Security Income and means-tested cash assistance (e.g. Temporary Assistance for Needy Families), a definition that closely matches modified adjusted gross income (MAGI), the income definition used to assess eligibility for Medicaid under the Affordable Care Act. Due to data limitations, certain other types of income that are not included in MAGI (e.g. child support) could not be excluded from the income measure used, but any resulting biases are likely to be small. Families units were defined using an algorithm for defining "health insurance units" (HIUs) developed by State Health Access Data Assistance Center (SHADAC). A description of this algorithm and programs for implementing it are available from the SHADAC website.[21]

It is important to note that this approach has certain limitations. First, Medicaid coverage is only available to citizens and certain legal residents, and this approach makes no attempt to account for the fact that the ACS includes many ineligible non-citizens. Second, the method used to model pre-ACA Medicaid eligibility rules is somewhat crude, and more sophisticated methods might give better results. Notably, however, Kenney et al. (2012) handle both of these issues in more sophisticated ways and arrive at broadly similar estimates of the share of potential new enrollees falling in specified age and gender groups. Finally, individuals' propensity to actually enroll in Medicaid coverage may differ across age and gender groups; failing to account for these differing enrollment propensities could cause this approach to overstate or understate the number of individuals gaining coverage in each of these groups.

APPENDIX B: ESTIMATING EFFECTS ON FEDERAL OUTLAYS IF STATES EXPAND MEDICAID

The most important input into analyzing how State decisions to expand Medicaid affect total employment and overall economic activity is how each State's decision affects Federal outlays. CEA estimated these amounts in two steps. First, estimates from the Congressional Budget Office (CBO) were used to estimate the total change in Federal outlays if all states expanded Medicaid relative to if no states expanded the program. Second, CEA distributed that national total across States using HIPSM estimates. This appendix describes each step in greater detail.

Focusing first on the national totals, the net change in Federal outlays if all states elect to expand Medicaid consists of two components: (1) an increase in Federal outlays reflecting additional spending on Medicaid coverage; and (2) a reduction in Federal costs to provide premium tax credits and cost-sharing assistance. The second, offsetting, component reflects the fact that some individuals in families with incomes between 100 and 138 percent of the FPL will receive coverage through Medicaid if their State does expand the program and would instead obtain coverage through the Marketplace if their states does not expand Medicaid. CEA used CBO estimates to estimate the size of each of these two components in a scenario in which all States expanded Medicaid, relative to a scenario in which no States expanded Medicaid.

To estimate the direct effect on Federal Medicaid outlays, the starting point was CBO's March 2012 estimates of the effect of the Affordable Care Act's coverage expansion on Federal Medicaid spending (CBO 2012a). Because these estimates pre-date the Supreme Court's decision in *NFIB v. Sebelius*, they implicitly reflect the increase in Federal Medicaid outlays if all States expand the program.[22] CEA then adjusted these amounts to reflect changes in CBO's assumptions regarding per-enrollee Medicaid costs from CBO's March 2012 baseline to its April 2014 baseline (CBO 2014b).[23]

To estimate the offsetting savings on premium tax credits and cost-sharing assistance, CEA used CBO's estimate of how the Supreme Court's decision in *NFIB v. Sebelius* affected the costs of these programs (CBO 2012b). CBO estimated that the Supreme Court decision caused a $28 billion increase in Marketplace subsidy costs in fiscal year 2022. CBO also indicated that they assumed that two-thirds of the overall expansion population would live in States that declined to expand the Medicaid program for individuals between 100 and 138 percent of the FPL. This estimate implies that, if all States declined to expand the program, the reduction in premium tax credit and cost-sharing assistance costs would be 50 percent larger than the $28 billion referenced above, so CEA scaled up the $28 billion estimate accordingly. CEA then projected this fiscal year 2022 estimate back to the present by assuming it would grow in proportion to total Marketplace subsidy costs reported in CBO's March 2012 baseline. Finally, similar to the Medicaid estimates, the resulting stream of costs was adjusted for changes in per-enrollee subsidy costs from CBO's March 2012 baseline to its April 2014 baseline.24,25

To distribute these national amounts across states, CEA relied upon estimates from the Urban Institute's HIPSM (described in the main text). Specifically, incremental Medicaid outlays were distributed across States using HIPSM's State-by-State estimates of the incremental Medicaid outlays in 2016 if each State elects to expand coverage. The offsetting savings on premium tax credits and cost-sharing assistance were distributed using the State-specific difference between the increase in Medicaid enrollment and the increase in overall insurance coverage that occurs if that State expends Medicaid (once again, using estimates for 2016); this difference approximates the number of individuals who would switch from receiving coverage through the Marketplace to receiving coverage through Medicaid if the State expanded Medicaid.[26]

As a final note, for the purposes of using these estimates with the CEA multiplier model, it is necessary to convert the fiscal year estimates that result from the methodology described above to quarterly estimates. In doing so, CEA assumed that Medicaid and Marketplace outlays occurring during fiscal year 2014 will occur smoothly over the final three quarters of the fiscal year (consistent with the fact that the main coverage expansions under the Affordable Care Act took effect on January 1, 2014). In subsequent fiscal years, CEA assumed that outlays occurred smoothly over the fiscal year. While the actual time path of these outlays likely differs slightly from this assumed path, any error in he assumed path is likely to have very small effects on the overall conclusion of this analysis.

End Notes

[1] Children (and, in some States, pregnant women) are eligible for public insurance coverage through a related program, the Children's Health Insurance Program. Under the matching formula used for CHIP, the Federal government pays a higher share of the costs, averaging about 70 percent and ranging across States between 65 to 81 percent in fiscal year 2014.

[2] HIPSM finds that if all States expanded Medicaid, the increase in Medicaid enrollment would be 13 million, somewhat larger than the 10 million increase in the number of people with health insurance coverage. The increase in Medicaid enrollment is larger than the increase in insurance coverage primarily because some individuals with incomes between 100 percent of FPL and 138 percent of FPL would switch from receiving subsidized coverage through the Marketplaces to receiving coverage through Medicaid. The difference between the two estimates may also reflect some offsetting reduction in employer coverage.

[3] Connecticut, Maine, and North Dakota have not reported suitable enrollment data to CMS and are therefore not included in these totals. For details, see CMS' April 2014 Medicaid enrollment report (CMS 2014).

[4] Many individuals in the control group reported receiving all needed care because no care was necessary or because they were able to access care through other sources (including, for individuals who ultimately qualified for Medicaid through other eligibility pathways, Medicaid itself). Similarly, individuals with Medicaid coverage may report not receiving all needed care for a variety of reasons, including scheduling or transportation difficulties or challenges in identifying a suitable provider.

[5] In other work based on the OHIE, the authors find that Medicaid increases emergency room utilization (Taubman et al. 2014). This finding is not inconsistent with the increase in the probability that individuals had a usual source of clinic care; Medicaid may simultaneously increase access to primary care and make individuals more willing to make use of emergency rooms by protecting them from the high out-of-pocket costs that can come with such a visit. In addition, the finding that Medicaid increases emergency room utilization could change when looking over longer time periods (as enrollees build stronger relationships with their primary care physicians) or as a result of efforts to reform the health care delivery system, including efforts set in motion by the Affordable Care Act.

[6] Approximately half of States' Medicaid programs have undertaken "family planning expansions" under which they offer Medicaid coverage for family planning and related services, including pap smears, to some individuals who are not eligible for full Medicaid benefits (Guttmacher Institute 2014). In almost all such States, women who would gain eligibility for full Medicaid benefits if their State expands Medicaid under the Affordable Care Act could already have obtained coverage for pap smears via the State's family planning expansion.

Oregon had a family planning expansion in place during the OHIE under which eligibility extended up to 185 percent of the FPL (Sonfield, Alrich, and Benson Gold 2008); the State has since extended eligibility through 250 percent of the FPL (Guttmacher Institute 2014). The OHIE nevertheless found that gaining full Medicaid coverage increased pap smear utilization, perhaps because accessing such care is easier in the context of coverage for a comprehensive set of health care services. This suggests that expanding eligibility for full Medicaid benefits will increase pap smear utilization even in States with a family planning expansion in place. Expanding eligibility for full Medicaid benefits might be expected to have a larger effect in States without a family planning expansion, in which case the estimates in this report will understate the increases in those States. Similarly, State and local health departments provide certain screening services funded through federal grant programs or other sources. As with family planning expansions, the existence of such programs should not affect the conclusion that expanding eligibility for Medicaid would increase utilization of these services.

[7] The results presented by the OHIE reflect the effect of ever being on Medicaid during the study period, so not all individuals were enrolled in Medicaid for the full period over which the

change in utilization was measured. The effect of continuous Medicaid enrollment on the outcomes examined in this report would likely be larger, so these estimates are somewhat conservative.

[8] Using credit report data, the OHIE found no evidence of a reduction in the risk of bankruptcy over a follow-up period extending slightly more than one year from the date that lottery winners gained coverage, despite finding large improvements on other measures of financial strain. This difference in results could reflect the much longer follow-up period available to Gross and Notowidigdo. Alternatively, it could reflect differences in the types of Medicaid expansions under study; the expansions studied by Gross and Notowidigdo primarily affected children, while the expansion studied in the OHIE affected adults. The limited sample size available in the OHIE does not appear to explain the difference in results, as the difference between the estimate reported by the OHIE and the estimate reported by Gross and Notowidigdo approaches standard thresholds for statistical significance.

[9] As discussed below, this analysis does not use the OHIE to quantify the effects of Medicaid on physical health, as the relevant estimates are imprecise and not statistically different from zero. One concern with using the only the results from the OHIE that happen to be statistically significant is that, as the number of health outcomes under consideration rises, the probability that one will be statistically significant purely by chance rises as well, even if, in truth, Medicaid has no effect on any of these outcomes. In this case, focusing on the statistically significant estimates and disregarding the others can be misleading, a problem statisticians and econometricians refer to as the problem of "multiple comparisons."

One way of addressing this problem is to set a higher threshold for statistical significance when evaluating the results of multiple statistical tests. Using a standard method for computing that higher threshold (known as the "Bonferroni method") while taking into account that the study also examined effects on high blood pressure, cholesterol levels, and blood sugar control, the p-value for the estimated effect of Medicaid coverage on depression remains below 10 percent. This indicates that the OHIE's depression results are still unlikely to have arisen by chance, even after accounting for multiple comparisons.

[10] This approach likely slightly understates the actual reduction in depression as a result of expanding Medicaid. Kroenke et al. demonstrate that the screening tool used by the OHIE researchers also occasionally misses individuals who appear depressed in a clinical interview. To the extent that Medicaid also reduces depression in these individuals, the effects on the overall incidence of depression would be correspondingly larger.

[11] Note that, while this analysis focuses on calendar years through 2016 because these are most relevant for quantifying the short-run macroeconomic impacts, generous Federal support for States that elect to expand Medicaid would continue in subsequent years. Expanding Medicaid would thus remain an attractive proposition for States since they could continue to realize the direct benefits of expanded coverage at limited cost, even though States' decisions would no longer boost overall economic output.

[12] Reductions in families' exposure to out-of-pocket medical costs could boost current demand for goods and services through another channel by causing families to draw down "precautionary savings" that they have previously used to "self insure" against medical risk. In the simplest models, reductions in precautionary saving improve economic efficiency even in the long run since precautionary saving represents a high-cost way of protecting against risk, although more complicated models can lead to different conclusions. Gruber and Yelowitz (1999) provide some evidence that past Medicaid expansions have indeed reduced precautionary saving. Because the macroeconomic estimates presented in this

report do not account for effects of Medicaid expansions on precautionary saving, they are somewhat conservative.

[13] The Federal government is sharing in reductions in uncompensated care costs under the Affordable Care Act through statutory reductions in disproportionate share hospital (DSH) payments made via the Medicaid and Medicare programs. The reductions occur regardless of State decisions to expand Medicaid, so they are not relevant to the macroeconomic analysis undertaken here.

[14] This estimate is broadly consistent with uncompensated care estimates produced by HIPSM, the source for the coverage estimates used elsewhere in this report. The HIPSM estimates imply that State decisions to expand Medicaid will reduce overall uncompensated care costs by $183 billion over ten years, which is 28 percent of the $645 billion increase in net Federal outlays if all States expand the program that was estimated by HIPSM (Holahan et al. 2012). To the extent that reductions in uncompensated care represent a smaller share of the additional outlays, the macroeconomic effects of State decisions to expand Medicaid would be commensurately larger.

[15] The estimates produced by this model reflect the National effects on employment and economic activity resulting from each State's decision to expand Medicaid. While the benefits of each State's decision are likely to fall disproportionately in that State, because States are economically interconnected, some of those benefits will accrue to other States. For example, California has likely realized some economic benefits from Arizona's decision to expand the program and vice versa. States' decisions to expand Medicaid are, thus, important for the Nation as a whole, not just the States making those decisions.

[16] Because all of the State-by-State estimates use the same national multiplier model, these estimates do not account for difference in the extent to which there is slack in particular State labor markets. In general, this means that the job creation effects of States' Medicaid expansion decisions may be larger (and longer-lasting) in States with weaker labor markets and smaller (and shorter-lived) in States with stronger labor markets.

[17] Other portions of the Affordable Care Act's coverage expansion could drive increases in labor supply. For example, for individuals who were eligible for Medicaid before the Affordable Care Act, expanded Medicaid eligibility and the availability of Marketplace coverage means that they can now increase their labor supply without worrying that they will lose their health insurance coverage.

[18] This analysis uses the IPUMS-USA pre-processed extracts of the ACS for years 2010-2012 (Ruggles et al. 2010).

[19] Information on pre-ACA eligibility criteria are obtained from various reports produced by the Kaiser Family Foundation (Cohen Ross, et al. 2009; KFF 2009; KFF 2010). Pre-ACA eligibility criteria as those in effect in 2009; this approach is consistent with HIPSM, which also uses treats pre-ACA eligibility criteria as those in effect in 2009 (Holahan et al. 2012).

[20] This provides a crude way of excluding individuals who were eligible for Medicaid before the Affordable Care Act as a result via more expansive eligibility criteria that are applicable only to specific groups, like those with disabilities. These more detailed eligibility criteria are challenging to model in survey data.

[21] See http://www.shadac.org/publications/defining-family-studies-health

[22] In principle, these estimates also include Federal spending associated with previously eligible individuals who would newly enroll in Medicaid even if their State failed to expand the program, perhaps due to enhanced outreach associated with the Marketplaces. In practice, the number of such individuals is likely to be relatively small, so including them is unlikely to significantly affect the results of this analysis.

[23] Specifically, CEA used the percent change in CBO's projection of per-enrollee costs for children. While cost trends for children may differ slightly from those for adults, the changes in CBO's reported per-enrollee costs for adults incorporate changes in the composition of the Medicaid population caused by changes in States' decisions about whether or not to expand Medicaid. As such, they cannot be used to adjust for changes in underlying per-enrollee costs across different vintages of CBO's projections.

[24] CBO's per-enrollee subsidy estimates are for calendar years, while the outlay estimates are for fiscal years. In making this adjustment, CEA used an appropriate blend of the calendar year per-enrollee estimates to adjust each fiscal year estimate.

[25] The overall change in per-enrollee subsidy costs from CBO's March 2012 baseline to its April 2014 baseline may differ from the change in per-enrollee costs for a given enrollee with income between 100 and 138 percent of FPL, for several reasons. First, premium tax credit covers a larger share of the total premium for this group than for the average enrollee, and these individuals receive cost-sharing assistance, unlike some higher-income enrollees. In addition, some of the change in per-enrollee costs from CBO's March 2012 baseline to its April 2014 baseline may reflect compositional changes if individuals who were switched from Medicaid to the Marketplaces by the Supreme Court Decision differ from the typical Marketplace enrollee. The effect of these imperfections on the overall results of this analysis are likely to be quite small.

[26] This difference may also reflect some offsetting reduction in the number of individuals enrolled in employer coverage, but it appears that the reduction in Marketplace coverage is the primary component. In any case, the State-level outlay estimates are relatively insensitive to the precise method used to distribute the offsetting tax credit and cost-sharing assistance costs.

INDEX

A

B

C

G

H

I

J

L

M

N

O

P

Q

R

S

T

U

W